ITINGS

or before

NURSING IN EDUCATIONAL SETTINGS

MARION S. STREHLOW

BA, RGN, RHV, RHVT, AMIHE

*Education Officer, English National Board for
Nursing, Midwifery and Health Visiting*

Harper & Row, Publishers
London

Cambridge San Francisco
Mexico City São Paulo
New York Singapore
Philadelphia Sydney

Copyright © 1987 Marion S. Strehlow
All rights reserved

First published 1987

Harper & Row Ltd
28 Tavistock Street
London WC2E 7PN

British Library Cataloguing in Publication Data
Strehlow, Marion S.
  Nursing in educational settings.
  1. School nursing——England
  I. Title
  371.7'12   LB3407

ISBN 0–06–318389–7

Typeset by Inforum Ltd, Portsmouth
Printed and bound by Butler & Tanner Ltd, Frome and London

HvH - 44084(3)/6 .95. 5.90

CONTENTS

PREFACE AND ACKNOWLEDGEMENTS

This book is intended to provide a useful tool for school nurses, trained, in training or yet awaiting attendance at a course. It will, hopefully, stimulate debate and give ideas on how to cope with an uncertain future. The future of school nursing is considered directly and indirectly, and indications given on the means and methods needed to ascertain that school nursing takes its rightful place in the hierarchy of nursing, that it is perceived as a worthwhile professional activity and that the parameters and developments which may be needed to provide appropriate status are achieved.

Nurse managers or health service managers who are not nurses, but have responsibility for school health and nursing services, may find the book of interest. The organizers and teachers of courses for school nurses have long requested, nay demanded, a book of this nature.

The book should also prove of interest to teachers, doctors and others who are concerned with the health of the schoolchild as it will indicate to them what their expectations of an effective school health service can be, how the knowledge and skills of school nurses can enhance their activities and how they can enable school nurses to fulfil their role and functions.

Within this book school nurses are referred to as 'she', this does not indicate discrimination, but reflects the fact that at the present time all those known to be employed as school nurses are female. Should men become employed in this capacity, the principles and ideas expressed will apply equally, except where they refer specifically to women's roles. I apologise in advance for any inadvertant misnomer.

There may be some male health visitors who have a school nurse function, please accept that it is simpler to say 'she' than 's/he or they' and also accept the spirit in which this book is written.

The views expressed in this book do not necessarily represent the views of the organization for which the writer works.

ACKNOWLEDGEMENTS

Profound thanks to all those who helped and encouraged the production of this book, all those who asked when they would be able to see my often expressed ideas in writing, but not least the pioneers in textbooks for school nurses, Patricia Slack and Wanda Nash.

This volume would never have reached completion without the support and help of my husband, who constantly cajoled and also provided practical assistance, back-up facilities and unending patience. No 'thank yous' can express the debt I owe.

NURSES LEAD THE WAY

If the millions of nurses in a thousand different places articulate the same ideas and convictions, about primary health care, and come together as one force, then they could act as a powerhouse for change. I believe that such a change is coming, and that nurses around the globe, whose work touches each of us intimately, will greatly help to bring it about. The WHO will certainly support nurses in their efforts to become agents of change in the move towards health for all.

Dr Halfdan Mahlei
Director Genera
World Health Organizatior.
June 1985

Feature Paper No. 97

1
INTRODUCTION

Nursing in educational settings is becoming established after a patchy beginning and a century of spasmodic development. It is at last reaching its proper and rightful professional slot, despite current economic and social crises, or perhaps because of them. It seems timely therefore to review where we are going, and how we can get there in the most positive ways possible. This book aims to provide a review, in part by reflecting where we have come from, in part by looking at where we are now, but more importantly by considering present practices and theories, as well as aims, to enable appropriateness and, hopefully, to be one means towards a successful future.

The title took some heart searching. 'School Health' sounds too all-embracing and ambitious for a short text and already features in several titles (Thurmott, 1976; Whitmore, 1985); *School Nursing* is the one standard text already in existence (Slack, 1978) and still has valuable information to offer, but the present and future – including functions, roles and scope – have many challenges and stimulants and are broader than any of the previous documents suggest.

The parallel, some prefer to call it the umbrella, is called educational medicine – a positive move to give the diagnostic, rehabilitation and treatment aspects of health care during school life their rightful place in the context of medical practice. *Nursing in Educational Settings* seems most appropriate as the chosen title. It is not based on a medical model of care, or if and where such a model lingers, it is now moving towards a model of life and living based on the potential of each child. For the sake of brevity and readability the terms 'school nurse' and 'school nursing' have slipped into the text, but they are intended to be interpreted in this wider context. The title also described the all-embracing nature of the care required, i.e. physical, social, psychological and emotional, with the last gaining increasing importance.

The book is written at the instigation of many who have heard me talk on various occasions and who urged that my thoughts be put on paper, I therefore make no apologies for re-iterating the things I have stated at times during the past few years. If the following chapters stimulate debate, are thought-provoking or even cause a few raised eyebrows, the book has achieved one purpose. Some parts of the book will be based on my personal interpretation of the existing syllabus for courses, though they do not follow the order or sections of the syllabus (Syllabus CETHV, 1979; ENB, 1985). It is hoped therefore that the book will assist students and teachers on courses, remind those who have completed a programme and act as an *aide memoire* and help those whose pleasure it will be to revise the current syllabus and devise the course(s) of the future.

The intent of the book is to be a serious text, but there are no apologies to those who notice that interpretations are sometimes lighthearted. You may call it a coping mechanism if you wish; I prefer to regard it as healthy cynicism or scepticism.

It is exciting to be writing at the present time when all nursing is at the crossroads of new beginnings and when both challenges and opportunities have never been greater. The fact that all proposals for development have to be clearly defined, measured and proven worthwhile need not be detrimental. In the long term such parameters should produce more effective results.

There is an added spice to writing now. Ten years ago articles and books on school nursing were few and articles by school nurses were almost unheard of. The picture has changed dramatically. Last year saw the publication of a splendid book, written by three nurses *Health at School* (Nash *et al.*, 1985). Articles by and for nurses are becoming regular features in *Nursing* and other magazines (I am not referring to famous nurses such as Claire Rayner *et al.*), and school nurses are at last demonstrating their talents. I am convinced that much more talent is hidden as yet and look forward to increased publicity by and for school nurses. One untapped source of material are the splendid projects and studies produced by many school nurses attending courses, some of which deserve to be shared with colleagues and other professionals. This book is therefore likely to be the forerunner of other volumes.

I had intended to subtitle this introductory chapter 'Are school nurses needed in educational settings?' or even 'Are school nurses really necessary?' In writing the following chapters the two questions have been answered as foolish, and I hope that the chapters have added to proof positive of the school nurses' invaluable contribution to health care, as well as proving the need for more resources and opportunities to be given to the school nursing service. Some of the opportunities will only arise if the profession decides to argue and negotiate for them, and if it continues to develop and prove this development. The roles and functions described and detailed are likely to change and extend with time and place.

There is another hope within this text. The image of the school nurse and school nursing has not always been positive in the past. Going public, that is describing what is happening, what could and should happen and defining some parameters, should assist the image. Within the text there is a discussion of image and some suggestions on possible progress.

Finally, this book is a testament to my commitment to the development and progress of nursing in all educational settings, whether this is carried out by specialist school nurses, health visitors or the 'new' nurse who will emerge from the education and training of the future. It is a statement of my belief that only effective and efficient professional teams, and partnerships between professionals and parents in allegiance with the child, can achieve a move towards reaching health potential within the school-aged population. It also encapsulates my support for the World Health Organizations' aim of 'Health for All by the Year 2000' and some of their suggestions for success, and my whole-hearted commitment to achieving the goals set by the Alma Ata declaration. It is only a small pebble, but might it start the growth of a mighty mountain?

There have been constraints on space and time, and the content has had to be selective and sometimes sketchy; despite this, please enjoy it with me.

SUMMARY

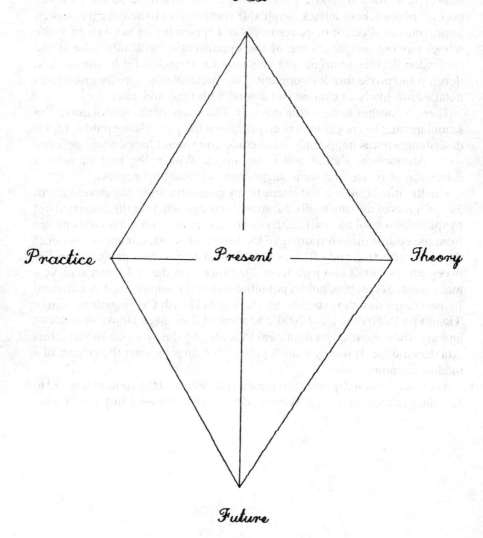

Past

Practice ← *Present* → *Theory*

Future

REFERENCES

Nash, W. *et al.* (1985) *Health at School*, Heinemann, London.
Slack, P. (1978) *School Nursing*, Ballière Tindall, Eastbourne.
Syllabus *Course in School Nursing*, CETHV (1979), ENB (1985).

Thurmott, P. (1976) *Health and the School Child*, Royal College of Nursing, London.

Whitmore, K. (1985) *Health Services in Schools – A New Look*, Spastics International Medical Publications, Blackwell Scientific Publications, Oxford.

2
AN HISTORICAL PERSPECTIVE

History, whether of nursing or any other topic, is fascinating. It lends itself to a multitude of interpretations; it can disguise or demonstrate any chosen bias and its major objectives – i.e. to illuminate the present and provide the means of enhanced and informed planning for the future – are often forgotten.

Additionally, history represents a time capsule, which can be short or long, clear or opaque, based on documented and proven data or guessed at by collating spurious evidence. It is really a distortion as today's events are already tomorrow's history; today's good or bad nursing practice produces either effective professional development and client care, or leaves a legacy – history – of problems such as the evidence found in reports of disasters, for example, inquiries into child deaths.

In some places, such as post-World War II East Germany, history lessons in school were a taboo subject because the education authorities had reached no decision at that stage as to the nature of recent history. The pupils enjoyed a grounding in Greek and Roman mythology and architecture, but left school with a knowledge gap about the first half of the twentieth century.

One detailed interpretation of the history of nursing has been presented by Rosemary White (1985) in her *History of Nursing*, an earlier summarized version was given by Anne Lamb (1977) in *Primary Health Nursing* with a most useful table of significant dates of special relevance to school nurses. More specialized histories, which reflect the practice, education, role and status of nursing in educational settings, are included by Wilkie (1979) and Battley (1985) in their History of the Council of the Education and Training of Health Visitors.

Current histories of community nursing, which includes school nursing, should incorporate the effects, policies and practices resulting from such documents as the Court Report (1977), the Warnock Report (1980), the Education Act 1981, and the Nurses, Midwives and Health Visitors Act 1979, and its subsequent Statutory Instruments. Of the last, the most important is Statutory Instrument 873 (Nurses, Midwives and Health Visitors Standing Order, 1983) which lays down the minimum competences required of any registered nurse, and the additional competences required of those with specialist qualifications.

The history currently being created includes developments of recent historical aspects, with additions of and adherence to – or deviation from – Codes of Conduct and Ethics (Code of Professional Conduct for the Nurse, Midwife and Health Visitor, 1984; Administration of Medicines, 1986).

Providing a framework for this historical development are the changes and policies affecting practice, the frequent changes within all service areas, especially the changes in health service management; government and local policies affecting health services; dramatic changes in educational policy and practice; local government provision such as social services; and the diffusion and development of voluntary services and agencies to meet a variety of needs. Just looming on the horizon, but gradually making their effects and implications felt, are such frameworks as the Health and Safety at Work, etc., Act, 1974, the Data Protection Act 1985, and the Police Evidence Act, 1986, each of which has an impact on how nurses, especially those working in public health or educational settings, can carry out their roles and functions.

The history of the future will be affected to a very great extent by the recommendations of the Cumberlege Committee which reported in May 1986 and made some significant proposals for nursing practice in the community: by the government's Green Paper on Primary Health Care (1986); and not least by the proposals of the United Kingdom Central Council (UKCC) for Nurses, Midwives and Health Visitors.

Project 2000 (UKCC, 1986) proposes major changes in nurse education in an attempt to provide realistic foundations for practice into the 1990s and the twenty-first century. It is based on an analysis of the situation which is likely to prevail in society as well as the trends which are likely to demand a different approach to professional practice.

The intention of this chapter is to chart the history of school nursing in a different way to that done before, and to see whether it provides a model which can be adapted for future use, or whether it may be desirable to note the past but consign it to its place and make a fresh beginning. Such a new start should have rapid progress as an inherent force, avoid the pitfalls of previous existences and have clear and defined aims or end products. The last, of course, may be affected in their turn by all or some of the factors which are crucial for any development. One of the facets of successful progress may have to be an improved use or even active manipulation of external factors, not just submissiveness to their influences. To date nurses have been, by and large, the manipulated and not the manipulators; future history may (hopefully) tell a different tale. The World Health Organization in one of its statements on how to achieve the international objective 'Health for All by the Year 2000' (WHO, 1978; 1985), has clearly perceived nurses as a major force with whom to be reckoned.

No historical perspective can ignore the influence of resources or economic provision. Despite philosophies to the contrary, community services remain underresourced. School nursing is one of the emergent Beauties among a range of Cinderellas.

INFANCY – VICTORIAN TIMES UNTIL THE NHS, 1948

The first school nurses were employed in cities which had acute problems among their school-aged populations such as infestations by vermin, infectious diseases, manifestations of poverty, diseases such as rickets and an inability to benefit from education except by the privileged few. School nurses were thought to be able to modify behaviour, teach attitudes and actions which would lead to better health and help to 'cure' the obvious ills. It is a sad fact that despite the best efforts of school nurses and other professionals from a range of disciplines and voluntary societies, the same problems are still found in present-day conurbations, with the addition of new ones. Environmental health, housing, income and availability of treatments have to support the preventive role of school nurses.

The abysmal state of health of the male population when required to serve in the Boer War served to alert the authorities of that time that all was not well, but it needed World War I to achieve full recognition of the value of early intervention if there was to be a human force ready and able to take action. After the war, children became precious as the investment for the future, so many adult males having died, that greater care was urged for their well being.

Those employed as school nurses in the early days were mainly mature women with variable backgrounds and experiences. For many years they remained few in number as they did not fit easily into any patterns of private or insurance-based health care, nor was it easy for public health service administrators – mainly Medical Officers of Health – to persuade local government committees to expend money on an unknown quantity with uncertain outcomes.

Roles and functions were locally determined, but generally covered basic needs of schoolchildren, including attempts to stimulate their development, and to encourage parents to send their children to school and to do so adequately clothed, shod and fed. The development of nursing in schools was accompanied by availability, at first patchy then more generally, of school milk and meals, thus enabling inadequate diets to be supplemented. Voluntary societies and welfare officers helped in the provision of clothing and shoes, and on-site treatment centres for minor ailments and dressings of sores became the norm.

Suspicion

There was considerable suspicion of education for all. The pre-Victorian and Victorian fear of an educated work-force lingered, and yet many parents were keen to see their children benefit from education and give them the chance of greater opportunities. It look a long time to realize that educational potential cannot be reached if basic needs, such as cold and hunger, are not satisfied first. The education system was very formally constituted and the introduction of a new element, an outsider such as a nurse, not always welcome.

Sending children to school clothed and shod was a real problem for many families. Apocryphal stories abound of children in families attending on a rota basis, each wearing the same pair of shoes in turn. Nurses, even then, were expert at organizing resources by a variety of means.

Nurses' job descriptions varied, but all had an element of treating minor ailments. The school nurses' normal week would include onslaughts on vermin, scabies, persistent sores, abrasions and often long-term treatment of limbs which had been broken and not properly set or healed. Assessment of health needs was an aim, and referral for appropriate treatment was attempted, though this was not always available, but both often took second place to dealing with minor and major crises.

Outbreaks of infectious diseases were common and one major task was related to disease control and prevention of the spread of infection. With the increasing availability of immunization and vaccination, and the changes in the nature of some disease-causing organisms, such as the decreasing virulence of scarlatina, these activities diminished and became spasmodic. Outbreaks of major infectious diseases among children in the United Kingdom are now comparatively rare, but they still occur and require continued vigilance by all those involved in the care of children.

The last major diphtheria outbreak in a populous part of London was in 1960/61 when one child died, several were infected and had to receive treatment in special hospital units and some unimmunized adults were also found to be ill. The school nurse was responsible for daily throat swab taking of all classmates, siblings and friends until at least three negatives had been obtained for each person.

The swabs had to be transported for analysis by the nurse (by bicycle) and many explanations given to anxious parents and teachers. Attendance at immunization sessions tripled for many weeks and Schick tests had to be applied to those whose boosters were overdue or where the record was incomplete.

The current meningitis outbreak in Gloucestershire, which is involving many health care workers, but places great onus on school nurses.

The above example is from personal experience and is on a minimal scale to the outbreaks which were current during the infancy of school nursing. One can now look back with wry amusement or horror at the extent of crisis work, and at the sad fact that many of the staff involved in dealing with minor or major epidemics were themselves unprotected or unimmunized at the time – myself included – a situation which should not occur today.

Infestation with vermin was common place; today's still large infestation rate is minimal in comparison. It needs to be stressed that overcrowded and poor conditions as well as poor health status were major contributory factors. Over 50 per cent of the parents of schoolchildren had no indoor washing facilities, approximately 40 per cent had no running tap water and less than 25 per cent had access to hot water. All the basic ingredients for infestation were therefore present.

The advantage was that nurses were saved from boredom by the variety of vermin – not just super-louse. Fleas, bed-bugs and ticks are just a few old friends. All still exist and occasionally make their presence known. At the time under discussion they added to morbidity by causing sores, inflammation of infested parts and sometimes general debility.

Bed-bugs don't like the light and only their bites were evidence for the nurse. However their presence leaves a distinct smell (like stale blood) and once encountered is never forgotten. Attendance at central cleansing stations and fumigation of the home were means of eradication. Some clinic sessions were marked by the variety of smells – the fumigant resisting all attempts at disguise.

School nurses of this early period had little or no formal training: some were registered nurses, some received in-service instruction, some picked ideas up as they went along. Perhaps this is the root cause of the slowness of achieving results or recognition.

Many of these pioneers worked part-time and suffered all the disadvantages of being unqualified, dominated by medical officers, usually male, and accountable to them, and being perceived as members of an all-female and therefore secondary group.

The image of the school nurse as an able and worthwhile practitioner was slow to emerge and be recognized and belongs to the period of adolescence of the service.

ADOLESCENCE – 1948 TO 1975

When the National Health Service was established in 1948 (NHS Act, 1946) provision was made for nursing care in community settings, including schools. However, the responsibility for providing this care was vested in local authorities under a tripartite system of health care. This created not only a division between various facets of the health service but also variable lines of accountability. It gave opportunity for community and preventive services, including those of health education and school health, to become pro-active and firmly rooted in the social settings in which they were provided.

The split within the nursing profession was amply compensated for by burgeoning working relationships with other caring professionals in the community. Nurses working in educational settings became close colleagues and allies with a range of workers, such as social workers, child care officers, education welfare officers, environmental health officers and school medical officers. They liaised with other nurses and health visitors working in the community, and with hospitals when children needed specialist treatments. They became responsible for encouraging high immunization up-takes, for health checks during school life, and for informing parents, teachers and general medical practitioners of the possible need for action.

In 1956 the Jameson Report reviewed community nursing services and confirmed the requirements of, for example, the Education Act 1944, stating that all nurses working in educational settings should be qualified as health visitors. This was in essence to protect pupils, especially females, but also to avoid a further split in a relatively small professional group, to enable all nurses to have adequate preparation and training, to avoid differences in status, salary and conditions of service. The government of the day accepted the Jameson recommendations in principle, but failed to act upon them. This nominal acceptance has never been rescinded, and remains theoretically valid.

The theme of school health was developed in the Cohen Report of 1964, which made health education a distinct nursing responsibility, with emphasis on health education at the receptive age, i.e. during school years.

Provision of nursing care in schools became diffuse, and local authorities developed services according to perceived needs, philosophies and resources. Some school health care was provided by effective teams of doctors and nurses; some by school nurses with access of referral to doctors and other agencies; some by health visitors, who often gave it low priority ratings within the context of their heavy and general case-loads; and some was provided by totally unqualified staff. To add to the confusion and profusion, some nurses were employed within the local authority health departments, whereas others were employed by the local education authority. School nurses were also employed directly by residential and private schools, as well as by voluntary societies running schools for children with special needs.

The result was that school nursing and school nurses did not receive full recognition of their potential and skills. Many nurses were in fact carrying out tasks which bore little relation to nursing or health care of any sort. Examples, which will remain anonymous, exist of school nurses providing a back-up service for school secretaries by doing duplicating of materials and other non-skilled tasks; of nurses acting as assistants at medical and other sessions without providing their particular input of knowledge and skill; and of school nurses being used to supplement community care for elderly clients and other groups.

Fertile years

There were local authorities who took their responsibility towards the school-aged population very seriously and established teams of nurses who led the way in providing effective health care, covering all phases of school life. The 1960s and 1970s were fertile years for change and development. All nurses employed to provide school health care were qualified nurses. It was recognized that adequate services could not be expected of those whose knowledge and skills were limited by lack of any basic education or training. The nursing qualifications varied and included state registered nurses, (SRNs), registered sick children's nurses (RSCNs), state enrolled nurses (SENs) and health visitors (HVs). It took some years to achieve this, as unqualified staff who had proved capable worked their way towards natural retirement.

The employment and deployment of trained staff produced not only an improved service, but led to ideas being promulgated and gradually implemented. There was a move for nurses to undertake comprehensive developmental checks, to carry out a range of assessment procedures, to take responsibility for hearing and vision testing and to provide a range of health education on formal and informal bases.

Gradually, school nurses gained confidence in their own abilities and began to take an interest in the wider professional arena. The first school nurses' groups were formed, and the School Nurses Forum of the Royal College of Nursing and the School Nurses Group of the Health Visitors Association began to make their voices heard.

As the nurses' confidence grew, so others' confidence in them reflected the new-found image. The 1970s saw close scrutiny of job descriptions and a gradual move towards a clearer job definition. Management structures started to include persons responsible for the development of this service in particular, and leaders with the expertise and interest to develop school nursing skills. In-service training programmes were developed in some places. The late Mrs Beryl Gettings of East Berkshire, and later Nursing Officer, Home and Health Department, Scotland, was an example of a nurse manager who developed both service and training.

Reorganization

In 1974 a major event took place affecting all nurses working in the community. The tripartite health service, consisting of hospital, general medical practitioner and local authority health services became a bipartite system (NHS Act, 1974). All local authority health services were amalgamated with hospital and other health services. The change was profound as it coincided with local authority boundary changes and produced 14 new health service Regions. New area and district health authorities were established within each health region, with revised management teams. With few exceptions school nurses were aligned to the community health services of the district, and based in health centres, clinics or other health authority premises. One aim of the changed bases for working was to facilitate teamwork with others also involved with the health care of children. The overall responsibility for child health remained vested at Area level, usually in the person of the Area Nurse/Child Health who, however, had variable management functions. She was usually instrumental in the selection of staff for employment and training.

Whilst the official date of change was 1974 (NHS Reorganization Act, 1973), in many parts of the country the change took months or years to come into effect, and some of it was accomplished very near to the next major upheaval, which is considered under the next heading.

For some nurses the situation became very complex. Not only were they subject to the changes affecting every employee, they also had to opt for a choice of employer if their authorities' boundaries had been amended; those who had completed some years of full-time service had to consider whether to transfer with existing or to accept new conditions of service. Nurses who had been employed by the education authority faced an even bigger dilemma, in that their choice included change of employing authority with all its implications. The majority opted to join their nursing colleagues in the health service. The most positive side of all these rapid changes was that nurses became aware of political actions and their effects, and it strengthened professional unity and development.

ADULTHOOD – 1975 TO 1986

The major changes of the early and middle 1970s were signs of the accelerated rate of change which set a trend which continues to the present day. The only certainty in today's working world is that there will be change, and that this is likely to occur rapidly and repeatedly.

There were five significant events relevant to school nursing which happened during the late 1970s. First, the publication of the County Report (1977) which described the needs of schoolchildren and recommended how these should be met. The government welcomed the report, but not all of its recommendations. Some action has resulted, but full implementation appears unlikely.

Second, the publication of the Warnock Report (1980) suggested how the needs of all schoolchildren, especially those with special needs, could and should be met. The reports' recommendations enhanced the role of the school nurse, and gave her extended responsibilities. In fact this report resulted in far-reaching actions. It was followed by a new Education Act (HMSO, 1981). The outcome most relevant to nursing practice is the establishment of multidisciplinary teams for the assessment of special need. The nurse responsible for the management of the school nursing services has to ensure that appropriate reports are submitted at the right time and place. School nurses have to write and submit reports on 'their' children. The first is the 'designated' nurse, in legal terms, the second is the 'named' nurse. In practice this has meant that each school has to know who the named nurse is, and how she can be reached at all times. In most districts this has extended the nurses' role, but some nurses are still expected to be responsible for far too large a population. The lines of accountability have become clearer as the designated nurse has the major responsibility and should take note of unsolicited reports as well as requested ones.

There are four other elements to the 1981 Act which directly affect school nurses:

1. They can initiate action, and in fact they are expected to initiate action as part of their function.
2. There is a requirement for regular reassessment of any child found to have special needs and the implication that no decision is in perpetuity.
3. Assessment can be requested at any age – from birth to school-leaving – and by any responsible adult, including nurses, teachers, parents and other interested parties.
4. Assessment records and the resulting decisions have to be communicated to parents or guardians, thus giving the ideal of working in partnership with parents a reality.

Most health authorities, together with the local education authority, have moved towards establishing the means and methods of meeting legal requirements; some patches have found implementation problematic and are still seeking success. At present the designated nurse is usually a person who also carries management and other child health responsibilities. There is nothing to prevent an employer designating any appropriately qualified member of staff to this function with all the explicit and implicit responsibilities.

Third, during 1978 the first approved training course for school nurses was established, to be followed by 21 others within the short period of three years. The training was a response to need and demand, and was approved following consultation with the profession and the Departments of Health of the four UK countries. The Council for the Education and Training of Health Visitors (CETHV) was invited to become the validating body, it being the only nursing organization which at that time had the relevant expertise. Negotiations resulted in a 12 week course, with certification upon successful completion. Proposals for a longer course were not acceptable to employers nor the DIISS. Between 1979 and 1986 16 to 20 courses ran every year and over 1,200 nurses completed the training. As well as enhancing knowledge and skills, the course provided the means to increase confidence, allow many hitherto isolated people to meet and gain from each other, and was perceived by many to improve status. The last was especially true of many teachers who finally accepted school nurses as qualified professionals. School nurses themselves appreciated the opportunity, but urged and are still urging that 12 weeks' training is insufficient, and that the programme should be extended. The approved training has been accepted by the UKCC as a recordable qualification, on the same basis as district nursing, teaching and a range of other courses. Funding for attendance at courses was and is at the discretion of the employing health authority, but for several years the Department of Health made funding available to health authorities specifically to second school nurses for training, thus stimulating this development.

The fourth significant event relevant to school nursing in the 1970s was that the Nurses, Midwives and Health Visitors Act (1979) changed the base-line for all nurses, and school nurses became voting members within the ambit of their professional framework. The Act was implemented in 1983, and its major effects are likely to form part of the future.

The fifth event encompassed the two major health service reorganizations within this short period. The first in 1982 again changed boundaries and some management structures; the second in 1984 fundamentally re-structured the management of the NHS and disbanded all area health authorities. While it is clear that the major effect will be at unit levels, the total results are only just emerging. The framework described above still exists, but with all the changes of roles and functions it is not clear in all places who carries which responsibility, nor what the lines of accountability are at present.

Additionally, this whole period has been one of economic recession and regression, and it has been difficult to negotiate resources for any develop-ment. Many authorities are suffering financial curtailments and are con-sidering every possible and impossible means of saving on expenditure. The in-word has become 'cost-effectiveness', and one spin-off is performance review of everyone and everything. Performance indicators are also much discussed, but to date few definitive statements have been made. It is significant that within the new management structures there is at least one person who carries the function of 'quality control', though at present each of these people appears to have different ideas of how to interpret the function, or its component parts.

Professional identity

The period of adulthood of school nursing has also been noteworthy for the development of a professional identity among school nurses. The formation of the Amalgamated School Nurses Association (ASNA) was one land-mark. It has provided study days and conferences attended by nurses from all parts of the United Kingdom, and also made contact with nurses from other countries, such as the USA and Scandinavia. More recently, ASNA has developed and published a quarterly journal (*ASNA Journal*) which is becoming increasingly interesting.

It is also noteworthy that school nurses and school nursing feature increasingly in other journals; the range of recent articles is too large to review here, but a selection is given in Appendix C.

The image, and hopefully the self-image, of school nurses has improved by all these means, leading to demonstrable expertise and greater recognition of the valuable contribution made to Primary Health Care by this group.

School nurses have generally accepted that they are accountable for their professional actions and decisions and that they may be asked to justify or describe them. They have also accepted that they are professional practitioners, who, while carrying out their own role are interdependent with other professionals. They are able to work in nursing teams, educational teams and form collegiate relationships with medical officers, teachers and others. All this is moving adolescence and adulthood of the profession into the era of maturity and towards the twenty-first century.

MATURITY – TOWARDS THE TWENTY-FIRST CENTURY

It is my belief that maturity represents fulfilment and serenity, not senescence. To consider moving to the next century is predicting the future and cannot be done with any accuracy. However, with the pointers given previously, and the discussion of extant proposals for future developments in the subsequent chapters, there are some factors which should form part of the history of the future:

1. Computerization of school health records is already developing. School nurses of the future will have to be familiar with the use of computers. They may develop their own programmes but most importantly they will know the facilities they should expect, and make use of both input and output services.
2. The majority of school nurses currently employed regard their post as a worthwhile job. Many work sessionally or part-time and are prepared to continue in their present sphere of work until they seek change. The recent past has seen appointments of nurse managers/school nursing. So far there is no school nurse in a teaching or research post, to my knowledge. Hopefully the future will see school nurses gaining job satisfaction by considering a career structure, both in terms of linking into existing structures and by creating new opportunities.
3. The recent past has seen school nurses taking advantage of available opportunities in some aspects of continuing education, such as attendance at refresher courses and the Health Education Certificate course. The future should see school nurses making improved use of all aspects of continuing education, including studies at undergraduate and postgraduate levels. To date, the range of relevant academic courses is small, and

there has been no demonstrable demand to increase this.

4. Some nurses are involved in professional activities and the future should bring an upsurge in active participation. Accounting and counting is the core of available evidence; until there are sufficient people actively engaged in promulgating the profession, it will remain limited in its scope and influence.

5. So far there are no male school nurses, except those among the 1 per cent of male health visitors who carry a school nursing function. Some local by-laws and paragraphs in early Education Acts which have never been repealed make the employment of males difficult, nor have men been attracted to apply for these posts. In some ways this has disadvantaged development; in future, consideration may have to be given as to whether the predominant femaleness could be turned to advantage.

6. A few school nurses have represented their group at district, regional and national levels. Very few have sought representation on national bodies, or have become involved with local or national politics. Emerging profes- sionalism should include and ensure greater representation on a range of bodies and organizations. This requires a commitment which transcends any job description and the limits of a prescribed working week. Such commitment is a necessary ingredient of a successful future.

The future is unlikely to be free of problems, new ones are bound to arise as old ones are solved. However, it presents a welcome challenge, and school nurses may find the recipe to maintain an indefinite but very long period of maturity before growing old gracefully.

SUMMARY

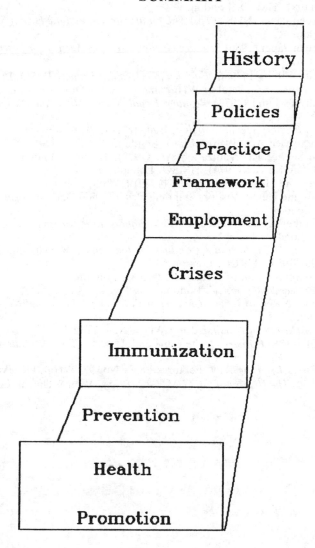

History

Policies

Practice

Framework

Employment

Crises

Immunization

Prevention

Health

Promotion

REFERENCES

Batley, N. (1985) *The History of CETHV 1975–1980*, English National Board, London.
Cohen Committee Report (1964) *Health Education*, HMSO, London.

Court Committee Report (1977) *Fit for the Future*, HMSO, London.
Education Act (1981) HMSO, London.
Government Green Paper, NHS (1970) *The Future Structure of the Health Service*, HMSO, London.
Government Green Paper (1986) *Primary Health Care – An Agenda for Discussion*, HMSO, London.
Jameson Committee Report (1956) *Enquiry into Health Visiting*, HMSO, London.
Joint Report by Director General of WHO and Executive Director of the United Nations Children's Fund (1978) *Primary Health Care: Alma-Ata Declaration*, Geneva.
Lamb, A. (1977) *Primary Health Nursing*, Ballière Tindall, Eastbourne.
National Health Service Act (1946) HMSO, London.
National Health Service Reorganization Act (1973), HMSO, London.
National Health Service Act (1974), HMSO, London.
Nurses, Midwives and Health Visitors Act (1979) HMSO, London.
Nurses, Midwives and Health Visitors Standing Order (1983) *Statutory Instruments 873*, HMSO, London.
Report of the Cumberlege Committee (1986) *Neighbourhood Nursing – A Focus for Care*, HMSO, London.
UKCC (1983) *Code of Professional Conduct for the Nurse, Midwife and Health Visitor* (2nd edn 1984), UKCC, London.
UKCC (1986) *Administration of Medicines*, UKCC, London.
UKCC (1986) *Project 2000*, UKCC, London.
Warnock Committee Report (1980) *Children with Special Educational Needs*. HMSO, London.
White, R. (1985) *History of Nursing*, John Wiley, New York.
WHO and UNCF (1978) *Primary Health Care*, and *ALMA-ATA Declaration*, Joint report.
WHO (1985) *Nurses Lead the Way*, Features Paper No. 97, WHO, Geneva.
Wilkie, E.E. (1979) *The History of CETHV (1962–1975)*, Allen & Unwin, London.

3
EDUCATIONAL SETTINGS

Educational settings can take many forms. They absorb all children from the age of five years, though some may enter earlier if they attend nursery school or a private preparatory school, up to compulsory school leaving age, which is currently 16 years. Many also complete further or higher education until the age of 21 or 22 years. The health care needs in each setting are likely to vary, but they do not diminish.

This chapter considers some of the formal educational settings, with their advantages and hazards, but it is stressed that the major settings, that is, home, neighbourhood and friends or social circle, have not been explored fully. It is being increasingly recognized, though not admitted by all those with vested interests, that whatever happens during the long school days and years, pales into insignificance in comparison with the influence of home and peer groups, playground or street corner. The most pervasive educator – life – does not have any one setting, but straddles them all.

NURSERIES AND NURSERY SCHOOLS

There are several opinions, each strongly held by their proponents, about becoming part of the educational system before one reaches the great age of five years. One faction maintains that the young child should be nurtured at home, that any teaching should be incidental as a component of development provided by parents or other full-time carers. This opinion gives little scope to negotiate nursery school entry according to the child's apparent need, either for the type of structured environment a nursery can provide or for those children who are eager to commence learning because they have the ability and curiosity or because they wish to emulate their siblings. There is also no acknowledgement within this thinking of the need of some mothers, either to have a welcome break from constant attendance on a child with its inherent nuisances and frustrations, nor the need to work so as to contribute to the family budget or to maintain adult contacts and sanity.

There are many children who live in restricted circumstances, for example in blocks of flats, and who have little opportunity to play safely, especially with sand or water, or with larger toys. There are also children who have minimal access to toys of any kind, and who could benefit from a range of stimulation.

Nurseries provide a reasonably safe environment for play and development, although no environment can be made completely safe with inquisitive children around. Nurseries also provide expert supervision to avoid dangers. Usually nurseries are based locally, a few are adjacent to the mothers' work place, and should not require an unreasonable amount of travelling. All nurseries have to be registered with the local authority (Nurseries and Child Minders Regulations, 1948; Local Authorities Social Services Act, 1970) and inspected regularly. They differ regarding the facilities they are able to provide and the number of children they are able to accept. In recent years the amount of nursery provision has diminished as local and education authority finance has become scarce. In many places, especially cities, nursery places have to be allocated to those in greatest need, such as single-parent families, children with special needs, or in the case of sudden crises in the family such as illness. While providing a safe haven, few nurseries do more than introduce the formality of education by attendance at regular times and days, occasional listening as a group to stories or music and some organized games and perhaps outings. However, they do provide the means by which children get used to sharing with others, leaving home and mother for short periods initially, and in some instances they provide the essential and sole means of learning social skills, such as handling cutlery, washing hands after having been to the toilet and basic good manners, saying please and thank you. It is fascinating to visit a nursery where most children are absorbed in their play, learning a tremendous amount by the toys and materials they are allowed to handle and the explanations they are given.

The second firmly held opinion, which is contradictory to the one described above, is that all children should have the opportunity for nursery-type education, that the benefits far outweigh any disadvantages, that it would ensure that all children are enabled to achieve more on school entry and that it makes the progression from infant to schoolchild easier. The growing movement of playgroups and mother and toddler groups is a step, providing a half-way house between spending infancy at home and being socialized with others.

Health needs

Children at nursery schools have health needs specific to their age group. They may require booster doses of immunizations, or in some instances have their original course completed. They may be subject to childhood illnesses such as measles, whooping cough and chicken pox. Some are very prone to throat and ear infections. They require adequate nutrition, suitable for the development of their fast-growing bodies, and some may need to be encouraged towards adequate sleeping patterns. Developmental assessments during infancy should have highlighted any specific problems and indicated any special care required. Assessments may have to be repeated to determine change, and hopefully improvements, but also to determine special needs. The aim of health care and health care plans during nursery life should be to ensure that the children are as healthy as possible and can therefore achieve their fullest potential during their years at school.

Nurseries present something of a dilemma for health care professionals, with the risk that children will not receive the care they deserve by falling between agency provisions. Health care of the infant and young child is the province of the health visitor, together with colleagues from other professions. Many health visitors will visit nurseries to see 'their' children, following their progress into the home. However, nurseries are provided by either the social service or education agencies and working relationships have to be negotiated at local level. Children with special needs may be the concern of many agencies. School nurses may have access to some nurseries, e.g. those which are on the same site as schools, and they have to agree roles and functions with colleagues. Most nurseries have qualified staff in attendance, such as nursery nurses, and day-to-day health care is their province as well as temporary guardianship. They are the most likely people to see parents on a regular basis and to be alerted to serious problems.

Some children are sent to nurseries for particular purposes, agreed between parents and professionals. One such group are children whose parents speak limited English and who may be disadvantaged if they enter school without language fluency. Another group are those whose parents have difficulties in providing the base-line for language development, for example, where parents have speech impediments or where they are prevented from communicating by other illnesses. An important group are children with minor handicaps, or rather with physical, mental, social or emotional disadvantages whose attendance at nursery may prevent these disadvantages turning into a handicap during later years. A small group of children are admitted for closer observation because assessments have demonstrated a deficiency, but the cause, extent or prognosis are not clear.

The role and functions of health care workers should be clearly defined in the latter instances.

PRIMARY SCHOOL SETTINGS

Infant/junior/primary schools are in reality an extension of nursery provision, initially facing much the same situation, but gradually providing more formal teaching input. The methods of teaching and learning in infant schools have changed dramatically in recent years. Children are exposed less to formalized tuition and are allowed to develop their knowledge and skills with guidance and expert help. They are encouraged to learn through exploration and experiment and by asking pertinent questions. The communication skills acquired in pre-school years can prove vitally important.

The health care workers' role, whether it be health visitor or school nurse, is one of guide and mentor. Health education can form an important part of the curriculum during these years. Children are curious about how their bodies work, about the way foods and other substances are absorbed and changed and a whole range of related topics. They are also receptive to ideas about hygiene, dental hygiene and other preventive health topics. Accident prevention is very important, as children run many risks during their exploratory phase. Accidents are not very frequent in schools, but road casualties increase as children gain independence in their route to school, and playground/park accidents become numerous. The nurse should be the major health educator. Taking account of her knowledge and expertise, she must be prepared to answer a range of challenging and frank questions. Additionally, she should support the teachers in their endeavours, by providing the information that helps them to teach health-related subjects, and most importantly answer health-related questions. Few teachers have the detailed knowledge to cover this subject and while they may not welcome intrusions into the classroom, they usually appreciate professional back-up. The nurse's role in all other health-related activities continues throughout this period.

There is one area which causes concern throughout school life, and that is child neglect, abuse and sexual abuse. Children of nursery and primary school age can be prone to abuse. Nurse and teacher should work together to investigate any suspicious signs and behaviour, and agree on the best action to take. This is a matter which involves the head of the school, as well as classroom teachers.

Some children attend private preparatory schools from the age of three or four until they are 10 or 12. They have the same health care needs as other children of their age-group, but right of access to private schools has to be negotiated individually. It may be essential to keep routine and regular contact with the parents of these children to ensure that their health needs are met.

Early school life has a few major crisis points, namely, initial school entry and transfer of school, as well as any period of prolonged absence or illness. Awareness of a potential crisis can prevent any substantial problems, and lead to action such as support and adequate, appropriate explanations which will minimize deleterious effects.

There is one particular topic which fascinates children within this age-group, namely death. They love the rituals surrounding death, but demonstrate their incomplete understanding by the fantasies they evolve. They are likely to ask very searching questions. Additionally, during this time many children first become aware of death, by losing a close relative, such as a grandparent, or a pet. The subject of death is a painful one for many adults to discuss, and nurses have been noticeably reluctant to get involved in any debate with teachers or children.

It would seem that nurses are ideally suited to talk with children about death, after all they have encountered it during their careers if not in their private lives. They are often ambivalent in their approach to the subject, and inclined to give vague answers to question. This is an understandable but unacceptable attitude. A change in attitude in dealing with questions and discussions of death is urgently required and each nurse will have to initiate this for herself so that inhibition becomes openness. This may mean admitting one's own fear of death or dying (a fear that recedes once acknowledged) and facing the fact that no one knows all the answers. Each nurse's beliefs may affect the responses given, but each nurse also has to acquire substantial awareness of a range of cultural and religious ideas related to the subject which may be very relevant to the child. The time needed to adjust one's approach to the subject will vary, but with conscious effort it should not take too long. A realistic approach should not be a morbid dwelling on the subject, but an open acceptance that death is a fact of life.

SENIOR SCHOOLS AND TEENAGERS

Senior school is a blanket title covering the range of school provision from 11 to 13 years and for the remainder of compulsory schooling up to the age of 16 years. The earlier age range is due to the variation of provision within education authorities, from grammar schools and some intermediate establishments in other places.

A division between grammar schools, entered by proof of ability or merit, and other secondary education provision used to be the norm. Comprehensive education became the policy and ideal during the late 1960s and 1970s (Robinson, 1968), but has never been fully achieved. There used to be additional specialist provision, for example technical education, which has now dwindled to minimal proportions. Specialist subjects were incorporated into the system of comprehensive schooling; it is not clear whether this move has been satisfactory. There are plans and proposals to strengthen the specialist or vocational elements of comprehensive education. Special schools for children with special needs are still in existence, but following the 1981 Education Act they are disappearing or changing their nature. They are considered separately in Chapter 4.

Some comprehensive schools were built during the boom of the 1970s and can provide a warm, light, airy and pleasant environment for their occupants. They have, however, been found to be less than perfect and all caring staff, including nurses, have to be vigilant about health and safety aspects. The school environment comes under the provision of the Health and Safety at Work, etc., Act, 1974 and school nurses have a responsibility to report any unsafe practice, especially in laboratories and workshop areas, or any recurring accident black spot. More recently, school nurses have had to be aware of the suitability of buildings for all pupils and should alert headteachers or their own senior officers to the special needs of some pupils in terms of adaptations needed to buildings.

A great number of pupils continue to be housed in elderly buildings, some of historical interest. It is difficult to ascertain safety aspects in these circumstances, but the same or a greater degree of vigilance is required. Additionally, it should be noted whether the building has deficits which constitute a health hazard, such as excessive dampness or inadequate lighting.

Medical rooms

Each school should have a medical room as specified in the original Education Acts, 1944 and 1948. This should be available to the nurse by prior arrangement, and should be adequate to carry out assessment procedures in a professional manner. Rooms which are not suitable for vision or hearing testing or which do not facilitate the accurate measurement of weight or height cannot be considered adequate for competent professional practice. In the past, medical rooms had all sorts of uses, and some nurses had problems in gaining access. Some schools had great pressures on space and found it unwise to leave a room available for periodic use; however, with the smaller number of pupils now in the system (there is reported to be a population drop for this age group), this no longer constitutes a valid argument. Nurses must be accountable for their professional practice (UKCC, 1983–86), and should firmly and clearly report inadequacies and negotiate improved conditions.

Another essential is space and facility to store records and other relevant materials. This might be in co-operation with the head-teacher who wishes to keep all records in one place, or following the policy of the health and education authorities. With the advent of computers, and computerization of school health records, this facility may not be needed, one central store being made accessible.

Additional to the range of public sector education provision, there is an increasing number of 'public' (which are really private, fee-paying), direct grant (which are really public) and private schools catering for pupils from all walks of life. They used to cater for the select few, but most now admit students on merit and at the recommendation of educational psychologists and other professionals. Schools catering for children from specific cultural or religious backgrounds complete the profusion or confusion; some of these are within the public sector and therefore follow 'normal' school regulations, others are private and make their own rules within the legal framework of the country.

Health needs

Whatever their physical environment, school-aged children have health needs. School nurses must discover these needs and the means to meet as many as possible, and to record and report those which cannot be met. They must also determine how many of these needs are individual and localized, and which are part of a pattern requiring attention at district, regional or national level.

It would fill a whole volume to discuss the health needs in detail, and especially their changes over time and circumstances, but a few indicators are given here and in Chapter 5.

'Normal' development

The primary need remains 'normal' development in order to reach adulthood in the best physical and psychological form, but in the meantime reaching maximum educational potential. Regular assessments, health surveys and health care interviews should assist in achieving this goal.

Another primary need remains adequate nutrition, though this constitutes one factor within development. Children and young people within this age group are no longer dependent on the food their parents or schools provide, since they visit tuck shops and other attractive paradises. Their nutrition may become distorted in consequence, and malnutrition, nutritional disorders and obesity can become realities. School meals used to ensure that each child had at least one meal per day, providing a high proportion of essential nutrients (one third of the recommended daily intake was specified by regulations). In many places such meals are no longer available and where school canteens are functional they often allow free choice by self-service, so not ensuring that nutritional balance occurs.

School milk used to be another nutritional support, but this is rarely found now at senior school levels. School nurses should assess the nutritional state of the children for which they have responsibility, and note any relevant trends. The cessation of school milk and meals is comparatively recent, and so existing evidence of effect on health status remains scarce. However, the emerging reports from the National Dairy Council give cause for concern. Health education has to be the major means of affecting success, and creating the attitudes and knowledge base which will achieve healthy adulthood despite inherent problems. Specific conditions such as anorexia nervosa, a self-induced illness caused by excessive slimming with psychological undercurrents, belong to discussions of ill-health, not school health.

Schoolchildren, especially as they reach their teens and adolescence, need to know that they are respected. They become resentful of patronage, and wish to be recognized as individuals – people. The nurse can assist in this by explaining to them all matters related to health and assessment as well as involving them in making plans for their own healthy future. Some nurses have found that if they make an unwritten contract with the young person to take certain actions, e.g. to avoid fatty foods, this has beneficial outcomes.

Growing up

Many schoolchildren are caught unawares by the approach of adolescence, and are very surprised and sometimes shocked at the developments to which they are subject. They start believing that they are abnormal, when in fact they are just reaching average milestones. Nurses may have to explain the process of maturation, the nature of adolescent development and the different phases each youngster is likely to experience. Such explanations may be rooted in the practical, for example, in how to cope with the practicalities of menstruation. Other concerns may have their base in biological factors, for example, in how hormones cause changes in voice and physique, or emotional aspects, e.g. in mood swings. The nurse's role should incorporate guidance to the youngster as to how these can be accommodated and so reduce conflict with parents, teachers and others.

A great anxiety among teenagers is their relationship with the opposite sex. They become anxious if they do not feel attracted or attractive, and at least as anxious about sexual relationships. There is a mixture of wishing to be 'grown-up' and resenting the pressures of peer groups and significant outsiders. School nurses can help young people to understand their reactions to their own bodies and to the attraction and repulsion of others, and lead them to recognize the values of loving relationships rather than sexual acts. They can help young people decide what is appropriate for them, and how to be their own guide, rather than submit to pressures. They can explain sexual development and relationships, and perhaps emphasize that there is no one right action appropriate for every person.

Teenage pregnancy

One problem which occurs in many senior school settings, in some at epidemic proportions, is teenage pregnancy. This certainly constitutes a health care dilemma, which involves not only the school nurse and teachers, but the specialist and social worker, not to mention the parents. The nature of much teenage pregnancy has changed. It used to be mainly due to 'accident' or ignorance, neither of which should exist with effective health education. In many places it has become a status symbol and the means of avoiding the demoralising non-person effect of becoming an unemployed female on leaving school with nothing to call her own. This has become intensified by the open acknowledgement of paternity by young teenage fathers and pride in their achievement, though with no means of providing for mother or child, nor very often the desire to establish permanent relationships. Another factor is the collusion of many very young grandmothers who are thrilled to have a baby within the family, without the problem of undergoing pregnancy or labour. The school nurse has to cope with the immediate health problems and risks, but she must also educate towards the responsibility an infant represents, and the situation which will arise as this baby grows and the young mother suddenly finds her life restricted.

Substance abuse

Drug, alcohol and solvent abuses are part of everyday concerns in many settings. The school nurse is not the only agent involved in coping with the dilemmas created by these abuses, nor is she the expert who provides rehabilitation or treatment. However, she is likely to be the one who notices the problem, recognizes the symptoms and refers to the appropriate agency for further action. She may be involved with the head-teacher and others, in attempting to prevent abuse becoming common place in the school, and to prevent individual addictions. Smoking is one addiction, and has to be treated in the same way, although the harmful effects may manifest much later and are therefore more difficult to demonstrate despite the vast range of media publicity.

The school nurse should be alerted to new methods of 'getting a kick'; substances abused are changing rapidly, and many teenagers will try a range of materials. The school nurse may also have a public or citizenship duty in notifying the authorities who have the power to restrict sales, or enforce legislation for restricted sales of certain goods.

Mental health

Mental health has suffered due to increased stresses among young people in recent years. Adolescence has always been a stressful period, but the prospect of an unemployed future or of few means of advancement or adventure has made this an increased health problem. The underlying causes are outside the control of any one person, even a school nurse, but her listening, supporting and counselling skills are likely to be in demand to try to prevent disastrous outcomes.

Violence

Children are growing up in an increasingly violent society, with violence at all levels, within the family, neighbourhood and wider environment. They are exposed to reports of violence on news bulletins and in papers, and within their entertainments. This has become a fact of life. School nurses may be instrumental in defusing potentially violent situations, but above all they can help by being non-judgemental, posing pertinent questions during health education sessions, and by demonstrating that aggressive behaviour is not scaring to them, nor will they become aggressive in their role. They can be an example of the substantial difference between positive assertive behaviour and negative violence. Assertiveness is essential to success (Townsend, 1985); violence affects the perpetrator as much as the victim.

One aspect of violence which worries many practitioners, among them school nurses, is verbal abuse. This is not uncommon, and can often be defused quite speedily. It is least effective if ignored, but it is important that the nurse learns not to show shock or disgust and that she desists from retaliation. It does help if one's vocabulary is attuned to understanding the abuse being produced. Working with a teenage population one has to learn a new language every few months, or at least new useage of the same language.

Young people appear to demonstrate little respect for authority figures. They act 'cool' towards teachers, parents and any person they perceive as representing authority. This is sometimes a defence mechanism and is overcome by building up mutual trust and an effective relationship. Respect has to be earned and maintained – the concept of role model, rather than authority figure, of mentor and guide, rather than instructor, is a helpful tool.

These are just some of the health-related needs which will be encountered by school nurses, and are additional to all the needs and occurrences which persist through school life, such as infections, accidents, assessments, and severe and minor ailments.

One dilemma not yet mentioned, but which forms part of any educational setting, is the fact that education is geared towards academic success and is examination-based. The intrusion of health education or health care procedures can form an uneasy alliance. Recognition of health needs is only the first step. Implementing action is the difficult second step, with follow-through of activities as the third and vital step. Evaluation of outcomes then completes the process.

FURTHER AND HIGHER EDUCATION

The settings in this arena vary at least as much as those in the secondary sector; the whole is described as 'tertiary' education. It is debatable whether students continuing their education require services from school nurses, health visitors, counsellors or occupational health nurses. In some instances they may require attention from all these professionals and others; in other instances they may believe themselves self-sufficient.

What is certain is that sixth form colleges providing courses for the 16 to 18 year age-group are administered by local education authorities and subject to the same regulations as the schools within that authority. The students are of an age when they can no longer be compelled to attend school or college, and they are therefore present with mixed motivations. The reasons vary, but there are three main ones:

1. Desire or coercion to take GCE A level studies or their equivalent, and in some instances to repeat examinations at O or A levels in which they were not successful at other institutions.

2. To commence vocational training by following courses giving foundations for work in industry or commerce. Pre-nursing courses are also provided by some sixth-form colleges.
3. To fill a gap between school and work while waiting for decisions about the future. It is not clear whether this group attends to alleviate their inherent boredom or whether they attend with the intention of being bored. Either way, teachers or nurses trying to achieve some motivation or create interest have a very onerous task.

Obviously, this group have health needs. Some are those unresolved from school years, some the 'normal' or exacerbated ones of adolescence, while others are created by the present style of living in a teenage society. The problems associated with excess intakes of alcohol, heavy smoking, accidents (they are now legally able to ride scooters and motorcycles and most eagerly await the birthday which allows them access to car driving), abuse of drugs and solvents are all part of the pattern. The percentage of students involved in this variety of abuses is likely to be larger than that found at secondary level, especially in relation to their total number, but they are much less likely to be noticed as the system is a less formal one.

Significantly, this age-group is likely to ignore 'healthy eating', either over-indulging or missing out on essential meals and nutrition. Apart from those young people with overt disorders, the damage is likely to manifest itself during adulthood, not at this stage, and is therefore difficult to combat.

This age-group is also prone to depression and suicidal tendencies are not uncommon. Where chances of obtaining employment are low, and where opportunities for continuing education are scarce or inappropriate, the number of youngsters with acute depression multiplies. Often this manifests differently to depression in mature adults, some of the symptoms being aggression, violence or apathy.

Young people remain prone to infections, but the predominating diseases change from those of childhood. Sexually transmitted diseases become a real hazard.

Teenage pregnancy continues to provide one health hazard, in some districts in epidemic proportions. There is some evidence that an increasing percentage of teenage pregnancy, especially among the younger teenagers, is the result of incest or sexual abuse (National Society for the Prevention of Cruelty to Children, 1983, 1984, 1985; National Children's Home, 1984, 1985, annual reports).

Not proven, but giving rise to concern, is the fear of permanent hearing loss due to exposure to continuous noise. Noise levels are often high, with cars, aeroplanes, thinly built houses and flats, and high population levels being some contributors. Teenagers are exposed to additional noises, by attendance at discos, by the constant wearing of 'personal stereos', and by continuous listening to or backgrounds of loud music. Assessments have shown that there is a definite hearing loss following attendance at a pop concert or disco, although in most instances this returned to normal measurements after one or two hours. The results of constant exposure to noise have not yet been accurately measured.

The same age-group of students who attend sixth-form colleges may alternatively opt to continue their education in colleges of Further or Higher Education. Here they are subject to regulations applicable to adults, i.e. they have to follow the exingencies of a course programme, not a strict timetable. They may continue in these institutions until the completion of their studies, up to and beyond the age of 21. They are joined by mature students, who may choose to commence their studies on a full- or part-time basis after they are established in a career or profession, and who usually are strongly motivated to be present either out of interest in the subject, or for career advancement. The health needs during this time become those of adults, often first-time parents. In some instances the health needs of school-age persist.

Most larger institutions of further and higher education have established student services, including medical, counselling and pastoral services. The role of the school nurse or health visitor becomes more tenuous. Her expertise and skills can best be utilized by providing back-up to the existing staff, by acting as a referral agent, and by providing the essential link between institution and home. Where services are not established, the health care worker may have to be instrumental in initiating services and providing coverage in the same way, though on a different level, as that provided for schools. The occupational health responsibility of school nurses continues to be valid.

Universities are part of the higher education set-up. The greatest difference in health needs is that created by the distance of the students from their home environment. Overtly, young people at university welcome the illusion of independence; in reality many experience additional stress.

OTHER SETTINGS

There are two other settings which cannot be ignored, and another important factor which should form part of any setting. The first of these, increasingly important, is the mass media. Young people are bombarded with information from television, films and videos, as well as papers, magazines and books. Many purport to be educational. The control of this flow of material is outside the ambit of the nursing profession, but school nurses should be actively involved in advising on programme development, monitoring the content of a range of literature and alerting the responsible authorities to material which is known to be harmful. Additionally, the material can form part of the health education component of the school nurse's contribution, either by demonstrating and counteracting inaccuracies or by using new and valuable items in her teaching materials. All this requires the nurse to be aware of recent research, its findings and applications and to be prepared to communicate at all levels.

The second important factor is that some children and young people have withdrawn from the formal education system and are being educated at home. This can occur at any age and be initiated by the child or parent. The educational content of home tuition is monitored by the education inspectorate, and must demonstrate a minimum level or standard, but health needs may not receive sufficient attention. The number of students spending their school days at home will vary greatly with time and place. It was very fashionable during the late 1970s and early 1980s in parts of the country, and has led to the formation of a few centres of 'alternative' education. Some of the most striking instances have received media coverage. Home tuition can be provided by parents, or parents can purchase relevant expertise. It is an interesting thought that a privileged few have in the past been educated at home by tutors – most of their children now attend schools, whereas some of those who have espoused causes of equality, etc., also argue or the freedom to be in total control of their children's education.

Lastly, the factor of importance in all these settings is how the nurse is perceived – her image. The school nurse should be able to present herself as an expert in health and child development, as authoritative but not authoritarian, as a constant in a changing world, a person who can be approached with confidence, in confidence, and above all a representative of 'authority' who is acceptable and who can be tolerated and respected.

SUMMARY

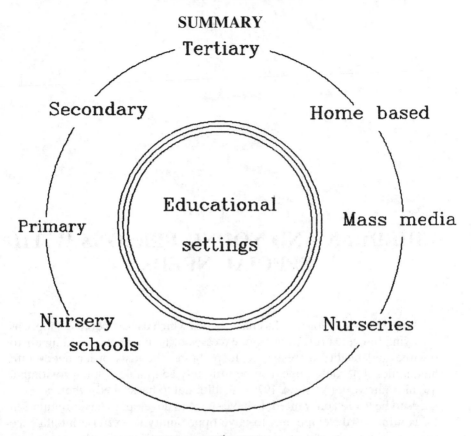

Tertiary

Secondary

Home based

Primary

Educational settings

Mass media

Nursery schools

Nurseries

REFERENCES

Education Act (1981) IIMSO, London.
Health and Safety at Work, etc., Act (1974) HMSO, London.
Local Authorities Social Services Act (1970) HMSO, London.
National Children's Home, (1984, 1985) Annual Reports, London.
National Dairy Council, *Nutritional Services, Quarterly Review*, NDC, London.
National Society for the Prevention of Cruelty to Children (1983, 1984, 1985) Annual Reports, London.
Nurseries and Child Minders Regulations (1948) HMSO, London.
Robinson, E. (1968) *The New Polytechnics*, Penguin Educational Special, London.
Townsend, A. (1985) *Assertiveness Training: A Handbook for Those Involved in Training*, FPA/NHSTA, London.
UKCC (1983–86) *Code(s) of Professional Conduct*, UKCC, London.

4
CHILDREN AND YOUNG PERSONS WITH SPECIAL NEEDS

Each person, young or old, has basic needs which can be defined simply as satisfying hunger, protecting from excesses of heat or cold, needing air to breathe and facility to rest and sleep. Some theorists order needs into hierarchies, but these appear to be infinitely adaptable, while providing a useful framework (Maslow, 1979). Additional to basic needs, there are the needs to be loved and wanted, to have space to develop, to have stimulation for continuous development, to have opportunity to exercise intelligence and to develop inherent mental capacities, and to exercise in play or leisure.

Basic needs
–
—
——
–Rest–
—and—
—sleep—
——Protect——
——from——
——excess——
——Satisfaction——
——of——
——hunger——
——Space and air——

Children's needs differ from those of adults by degree; they need to satisfy the basic ones, they need exercise to develop physically and mentally, but above all they thrive on the secondary needs of stimulation and curiosity. They need love in order to learn to give love, they need security to learn through play and exercise, and they need warmth and protection.

Potential

Carers and providers

—Rest and sleep—
——Exercise and play——
———Safe environment———
———Satisfaction of hunger———
——Need to be loved and wanted——
——Need for security and protection——
————Stimulation————
—Satisfaction of curiosity—
—Exercise intelligence—

Inhibiting factors

Positive factors

Special needs

Continuing development

Each child is born with learning potential, which may vary in extent and there may be inhibiting factors in reaching full potential. The aim of school life is to achieve the highest possible potential; all caring services, as well as parents and family, should contribute to this achievement. School nurses can make a significant contribution here and be instrumental in identifying children who have additional or special needs and who therefore may require special stimulants or a different kind of approach to fulfil their needs.

Children at schools have needs which are outside the remit of any health care worker, though they beg the question of when one ceases to perform as a professional of a particular discipline and acts according to the dictates of conscience and as a caring citizen. The range of these needs may be vast or small according to circumstances, but could include such issues as employment/unemployment, increasing or persistent poverty, overcrowding with potential health hazards to the whole community, and environmental factors such as air pollution or disposal of hazardous substances.

School nurses and their colleagues may not carry responsibility for a range of limiting factors, but should be able to contribute towards their alleviation or provide the help and support which allows potential to be reached despite inherent difficulties. These factors include hereditary diseases, acquired diseases or handicaps, the effects of violence in the family or society, and restricted circumstances such as low income or lack of parental supervision. The last is a factor of increasing importance, with high divorce rates and large numbers of single-parent families. The decision each professional has to make is the extent of involvement, the nature of involvement or commitment and the timing of any action. The art and practice of communication are vitally important to all caring contributions.

The range of needs among children is extensive, and educational settings can only meet a proportion of them. Where the environment is reaching the ideal, the proportion of met needs increases; however, it is unlikely to provide sufficient quantity and quality if the setting is deficient, as many are in reality. As a member of the educational team, the school nurse should be an active contributor to the determination and meeting of needs.

Some children have needs additional to the normal range, either through illness, handicap or disadvantage. The Warnock Report (1978) considers the special needs of school children in considerable detail; the Snowdon Report (1976) looks at the special needs of young persons and adults, especially the extended and continuing education needs of adolescents. It would be inappropriate to reiterate the statements already made in these documents, as they remain entirely valid, but the following paragraphs seek to consider some aspects of special needs which are so obvious that they are often forgotten or missed, and constitute some of the 'grey' areas in health care and educational provision.

THE CHANGING NATURE OF SPECIAL NEEDS

Special needs are not a static condition, but incur changes within any individual, and their development, their environment and circumstances. They must be assessed with great care; plans must be evolved to meet them, and reassessed after the initial implementation of the plan, followed by amendment or continuance of the original plan, with regular repetition of the cycle. This is in essence a process approach, though it need not be rooted in any particular process. Recording of the assessment findings, documenting the outline plan and details of implementation and the reassessment are important in determining progress or regression, and to judge the validity of the care provided. The recording system used may be succinct or extensive, traditional pen and paper or computerized, but it should be accurate and clear, so that it can be understood and, where appropriate, followed by all those involved in implementation.

The recording system may be one which is accessible to professionals only, but ideally and practically it should be shared with the person who is the subject of the assessment and plan, as well as by the parents or guardians. It should contain the individual's agreement to follow specified actions or activities, i.e. their partnership in the process.

The obvious special needs relate to handicapping conditions, be they physical, mental, social or emotional. Physical handicap used to be very common, varying in degree and often related to nutritional deficiencies, e.g. rickets. At times particular handicaps predominated, such as the children born during the 1950s and 1960s with deformed limbs due to their mothers taking the anti-nausea drug thalidomide while pregnant. At present, most physical handicaps are acquired through injury or accident, and the total number of children suffering from physical handicap has decreased dramatically.

The major causes of physical deformity are therefore preventable, and the school nurse's input should be significant. The second major category causing physical handicap is the outcome of disease. The school nurse is unlikely to affect the outcome of diseases such as cancer or kidney malfunction, but she can be instrumental in preventing the disastrous results of infectious diseases, such as measles with its subsequent hearing loss. She should also contribute to the eradication of certain diseases by implementing a full immunization programme, persuading and advising those who do not wish to take advantage of the available protection, and educating young people towards complete protection of their future families.

Special needs relating to mental handicap constitute a broad spectrum. The degree of handicap is variable, and can improve or deteriorate. It has been demonstrated by the work of the National Society for Mentally Handicapped People (MENCAP) and its research and practical application that few mentally handicapped children are ineducable. Each has the potential to achieve something, and will do this at a pace and to a degree relevant to their condition. Some children will require the kind of individualized attention which can only be provided in special institutions or schools; others will be able or enabled to cope in 'normal' settings.

The school nurse should be instrumental in ensuring that the potential is maximized. The care plan should include the type of stimulation and attention which may lead to progress and independence, and wherever possible prepare the young person to live as normal a life as possible. In instances of mental handicap, the school nurse's major contribution may be in helping teachers to understand and lead their 'normal' pupils towards understanding, to act as mediator if there is evidence or suspicion of bullying or teasing, to provide an interface between caring agencies and to ensure that appropriate stimulation and care is provided. School nurses working in special schools or institutions will extend their involvement in the health care of pupils, to meet the needs of their special clientele.

It is to be noted that the nature of mental handicap has changed, and appears to continue to change. Many conditions, such as German measles (rubella) during pregnancy, are now preventable. The main causes of mental handicap are genetically determined factors, trauma during pregnancy or birth, and injury during infancy and childhood, either accidental or non-accidental. It would appear possible to reduce the number of affected children still further, but figures given regarding the numbers of handicapped children and young people vary and no true record of incidence exists.

OTHER HEALTH FACTORS

School nurses have an additional responsibility in relation to mentally handicapped pupils. They should ensure that there are no other health factors which affect development and could be misinterpreted as being part of the mental handicap; that attention to other needs is not omitted by using the deficiency to explain all behaviours, actions or comments. There is mounting evidence that health care professionals are prone to ignore the basic and general human needs of mentally handicapped people, through ignoring or misinterpreting their sometimes unclear description or statement of need or difficulty. The latter is more likely to happen when, for whatever reason, the person is transferred from the environment with which he is familiar.

Emotional deprivation

In contrast to the diminishing numbers of young people with mental handicap, and the improvements which have occurred in preventing such conditions, emotional deprivation, resulting in special needs or handicap, is increasing in incidence. Love and security are basic needs of all children, but many children do not experience the receipt of love and are subject to frequent and rapid changes in environment, relationships and living conditions. These children are likely to suffer from emotional deprivation. It is noteworthy that emotional deprivation is not necessarily related to poverty, but can occur in any strata of society. Children who are deprived of the basic ingredients for development, love and security are likely to exhibit signs of disturbance in behaviour or growth patterns. They will have difficulties in establishing lasting and effective relationships and may have learning problems.

It has been demonstrated by effective intervention, such as that provided by the National Children's Home and other voluntary societies, that deprived children have been treated as mentally handicapped, when in fact their condition is amenable not only to improvement but also to alleviation. The behaviour exhibited may range from withdrawal to exhibitionism, from being too quiet to being violent, and may often be noticeable by swinging from one extreme to the other. The school nurse should be aware of the signs of such deprivation and should investigate, along with colleagues in the health and education teams, what action can be taken to help the child to overcome this potentially handicapping condition. If left, the handicap may persist into adulthood, leading to repetition of the cycle of deprivation. It would appear that a child who has not received love and attention has a poor self-image and will find difficulty in giving love. A child who is insecure will have problems in creating or recognizing a secure environment, leading to further emotional and practical difficulties.

Children who have been made insecure by neglect, intentional injury by a parent or guardian, shifting relationships, permanent loss through death or divorce, or victimization may carry the emotional scars through the whole of their lives, often resulting in mental illness in later life.

It has already been mentioned that suicide or suicide attempts are not uncommon among schoolchildren. It is not clear how much of the incidence of drug and solvent abuse is due to emotional needs which have not been met. In the context of emotional deprivation, a few issues require closer consideration.

VICTIMIZATION

Victimization is the first of these. It is becoming clearer, from reports of court cases and the case-lore built up by a variety of caring agencies, that some children are cast in the role of victim, even though they may have made no conscious contribution to this attitude. The strangest, but perhaps very human attitude, is the active dislike of a child who resembles an adult who has given cause for trouble. The dislike may be dormant in the parent or guardian, and relate to unexpressed feelings about in-laws, uncles, fathers or any permeating factor of their own past life. One-parent families may blame a child for their difficult conditions or for its resemblance to the missing partner. Some children have characteristics or features which are abhorrent to their carers, including school nurses, and others which are not acceptable to their peers. In any event they may suffer for something which they cannot alter.

Victimization can take many forms, from minor irritations to major neglect or abuse. The victims of overt abuse, whether physical, emotional or sexual, are easy to define by comparison, though all may suffer far-reaching, immediate or long-term consequences and have an emotional handicap as a result. The victimization described here is mainly an ill-defined entity, with no apparent rationale. Some children belonging to particular social, cultural or racial groups may also suffer victimization. While no less harmful, the cause of this type of victimization can be determined and gradually eliminated. It is often rooted in prejudice. Because victimization is a manifestation of some deep-rooted, and often unrecognized, source complete eradication takes considerable effort, skill and time; during the process, the best that can be offered to any child is protection and special care to mitigate the effects.

CHILD ABUSE, INCEST AND NEGLECT

Child abuse, incest and neglect are all issues of serious concern, which can result in a range of special needs and sometimes in handicap or death. Child abuse, or non-accidental injury, has been recognized as a definable syndrome since the late 1960s (Kempe and Kempe, 1978). Predictors and indicators have been developed which are applicable to families from the prenatal period onwards. Despite the increasing volume of reports, the latest being the report on the death of Jasmine Beckford (Brent Borough Council, 1986), and the increasing awareness of all those working with children, it would appear that prevention is still an unattainable goal. Crisis lines, e.g. the ones established nationwide by the National Children's Home, and following the BBCs Childwatch programme, have become available and do sterling work in coping with cries for help and attempting to prevent abusive activities.

Health care and social workers from many disciplines are acutely conscious of their responsibilities; neighbours and friends often initiate action and yet it would seem that the incidence is increasing. There is one school of thought which states that it is not an increasing incidence, but the fact that greater awareness has led to more notifications and actions being taken. It certainly is not a new phenomenon, but a very worrying one. All reports and documents demonstrate the need for effective communications to bridge the vast gaps in communication networks which continue to exist.

The school nurse may notice or be alerted to children who are being or have been abused. Any signs and suggestions must be investigated fully with accurate recording of assessments and actions. The first stage of action is usually a 'case conference', which can be called by any professional directly involved. The usual way for a school nurse to call such a conference is through her nurse manager or the 'designated' nurse within any health district. It is one responsibility of professional judgement whether to urge for very speedy action, or whether to attempt other measures in the first instance. In either case the decision and its rationale must be communicated to the nurse-manager, the head-teacher and the medical officer, who may also urge a distinct line of action.

Neglect is another difficult area. The evidence is confusing as to whether it is potentially harmful or whether it can actually stimulate intellectual development and create independence. Each instance has to be acted upon according to assessments and professional judgement. One guiding principle could be the risk to the child of deterioration in health, of lack of reaching milestones in development, or the social acceptability of children who have been neglected. The most common signs of neglect are malnourishment and lack of cleanliness. Other signs could include nonattendance at school, odd or changed behaviour and isolation or withdrawal from the peer group. It used to be thought that neglect was a symptom of abuse or a precursor to it, but this does not appear to be true. Children who suffer from lack of attention are usually out of the reach of the abuser, except in the sense of providing a safe environment. Many instances of neglect come to light when children are found to be alone at home in risky circumstances, when they are of an age that requires supervision.

Incest is an issue which is debated reluctantly in public since it is a very emotive situation. The evidence accruing from a variety of sources, including helping agencies, the NSPCC and the media, suggests that the problem is more widespread than previously thought. It would appear that incest can occur between father or uncle and daughter, mother and son, brother and sister or any variation of relationships. The greatest difficulty surrounding incest, in contrast to abuse or neglect, is that it is often based on a loving relationship, colluded by other members of the family, and that any alleviation of the situation must include the protection of the child or children and also a re-building of family relationships on different foundations. The removal of the 'offending' adult may only create further trauma. One aspect of vital importance is that the child who has had, or been subjected to, an incestuous relationship must be helped to adjust, so that he or she can form effective 'normal' relationships in later life. This requires special skills, and the school nurse's role may be that of referral agent, as well as support system.

The caring agencies in the United Kingdom are very aware of the difficult and extensive nature of the problems created by abuse, incest and neglect. It is little consolation that the problems are not confined to one country, but are recognized internationally. Almost every country which contributes to debates, conferences and documentation in any of the international arenas has identified that problems exist, that they are increasing, and that the means of combatting the dilemmas are as yet unclear.

Concerns have been expressed that the wide publication of pornographic literature, video and film materials of questionable or proven 'blue' quality and the international availability of such materials have contributed to the difficulties. There is also increasing international evidence that parents are colluding in the use of children for a variety of purposes, sometimes for economic reasons, and often because they cannot understand the propositions being presented or the pressures being applied. These parents may be totally unaware of the real use made of their children or the long-term consequences to them. School nurses may contribute to the evidence presented at national and international levels; however, their main concerns remain the well-being of the child. It is noteworthy that proposed legislation may strengthen the child protection role of health care workers, and that the American school nurse is already legally accountable as a child protection agent.

DISSONANCE

One special need that arises among young people and adolescents is overcoming dissonance with their elders and environment. The 'generation gap' has become a phrase used in many ways; it is a common reality between parents and their teenagers, teenagers and younger pupils or siblings and teenagers and society at large. It has been a reality in every generation, but because of mass communication it finds speedier and overt expression.

The exploratory phase of childhood turns into the adventurous phase of teenage and adolescence which is compounded by experimentation, idealism, disenchantment and the need to 'prove oneself'. Conceptually most teenagers are still unable to discern 'shades of grey', and consider that they are the first to have found an answer to any situation, either at home, in their neighbourhood or worldwide. They cannot yet conceive of many complexities, nor distinguish between proven facts and doubtful ideas. It is an exciting time when physical and mental development are not always in tandem, one outpacing the other, and when important decisions about the future have to be made. Some young people are caught up in examination fever, some fear the future and a lack of prospects, some wish to try new pastures, some wish to remain in their known and reasonably safe environment – nearly all experience the aches and pains of growing up. They are neither adults, though they may have adult bodies, nor children. They are partially or fully independent, and the adults around them expect both types of behaviour, i.e. childish and adult, without apparent rhyme or reason. The school nurse can make an important contribution in assisting the process of maturation, by explaining the turmoil being experienced, by answering health-related questions which arise frequently, and by providing a health education input which lays the foundations for adult independence and responsibilities.

MINORITY GROUPS

It is often claimed that children from minority groups, whether ethnic or religious, have special needs. This claim appears to be based on a doubtful premise. Children from all groups have the same fundamental needs. It may be necessary, and school nursing may be one facet of this, to ensure that membership of a particular group does not create disadvantage, that inclusion into school society is effective and that there are no additional health hazards resulting from membership of the group. Some groups have particular dietary regulations or are used to using dietary materials differently. It is important that this is interpreted in terms of the child's needs and adaptation to the climate of the UK. Often the parents or carers rather than the children need help because they would wish to avoid hazards and may not know how to adapt the materials to hand. Children may require additional protection from prejudice or misunderstanding, and some children may be disadvantaged by language difficulties. The school nurse's role is to assess the situation and take the appropriate action, for example to ascertain that children get extra tuition in language use, rather than be 'written off' as being of low ability. It is also essential that the measurement and assessment tools used by the nurse are appropriate for all groups.

MINOR ILLNESSES

A large area of special needs are caused by periodic ill-health, accidents and their results, convalescence and periods of rehabilitation. Many children do not reach their educational potential because they suffer repeatedly from minor illnesses. These illnesses are termed 'minor' because they do not require 'high-tech' treatment or expensive drug therapy and because they are often self-limiting. In developmental or educational terms they may cause major disadvantages, adversely affecting both, and being difficult to overcome. Children who have frequent heavy colds with subsequent catarrh may have temporary hearing loss, and although this is not deafness, it will limit the capability to benefit from educational input. Children who have recurrent sore throats may be limited in the contribution they can make to classroom activities and may therefore be regarded as 'backward'. Children who have persistent aches and pains, including toothache, can exhibit difficult behaviour. These children often cannot explain why they are behaving strangely nor is the cause easily recognized, unless they are subject to regular health surveys.

Some children may be absent from school so frequently through these 'minor' illnesses that educationally they become backward and suffer the resulting disadvantages. The whole arena of minor illnesses requires much more attention than it is currently accorded, and school nurses should be very active in ensuring that any disadvantages are minimized. This may be through alerting responsible authorities to adverse conditions which are an underlying cause of many illnesses, such as bad housing, and by negotiating appropriate treatment to shorten the effect of any ailment.

HOSPITAL ADMISSION

Breaks in attending school may be caused by hospital admissions, which are variable in length. In theory, any child admitted to hospital should still be in receipt of formal education, either by peripatetic teachers or through materials supplied and contact maintained with the child's school. In practice this system is haphazard; some hospitals have splendid teaching facilities, but most hospitalized children are divorced from their usual contacts. In instances where the child is discharged into home and community care within a short period of time this may not be of major importance, but it does become significant during convalescence. Unless the illness is severe and prolonged, few children stay as inpatients for lengthy periods; however, they may have to attend for treatment and outpatient appointments for a considerable time, causing more disruption to their education. The school nurse may have to provide the link between curative health agencies and school, advising the teachers on the volume of work that can be coped with and the level of response which can be expected from the child.

Additionally, a link may have to be forged between home and school, child, parents and school, and effective communications established and maintained between all concerned. The school nurse is one important part of the communication network.

It is also part of the nurse's role to ensure that repeated, legitimate absence does not lead to absenteeism without good cause, to school aversion or phobia, and that confidentiality about medical aspects of the absence is balanced with the need to avoid rumour and misinformation with resulting teasing or disadvantage. Where the illness has been caused by an accident, the school nurse may have to ensure that relevant treatment and therapy is carried out during school time, and deformities or lasting effects avoided or minimized. Some nurses may be skilled to provide some treatments, but often this means close communication with specialists and therapists. It is likely that the nurse will also be the communication link between child, school, parents and school medical officer, though the processing of written communications between medical agencies, such as hospital consultant, general medical practitioner and school medical officer vary in each instance.

INTEGRATION

It is government policy, formulated as a response to many groups with special interests, to encourage integration of children with special needs into normal schools. Most education authorities have accepted the principle of integration, but some have progressed more speedily towards implementation than others. There are a few very real difficulties to be overcome before complete integration can occur, apart from changing the attitudes of some parents, teachers and pupils. The first is that not all school buildings are suitably equipped to cope with differences, nor can they be easily adapted, even if the financial resources were available to do so. The second is that few teachers are trained to deal with pupils with special needs; some are even afraid of being responsible for such children. Their overriding concerns are that they already have more pupils in each class than they can effectively teach, and that they may have to attend to special needs to the detriment of the other pupils. There is also concern that those who can provide specialized tuition will not be available to support the classroom teachers.

Few question the underlying principle, but many feel that effective action needs to be supported by sufficient resources, including staff. The school nurse is likely to be the bridge upon whom successful integration depends: she may advise teachers about the conditions or handicap which causes a child to have special needs; she may advise about the drugs being used to control a condition, their storage and possible side-effects, such as sleepiness or drowsiness in the classroom; and she can advise on what can be realistically expected in general behaviour and performance.

Integration of pupils into the normal education system, while accepted by most as a desirable principle, has had some serious consequences, of which not all are equally beneficial. The first is the changed nature of the remaining special schools. Special schools were evolved to provide a protective and stimulating environment for children with different needs, and often specialized in particular types of need. The staff of those schools were competent in meeting the defined needs, and people of suitable calibre and interests were usually attracted to work there. In recent years many specialized special schools have closed, often quicker than the integration of children into the 'normal' system. The remaining establishments may be far distant from the child's home, creating great dilemmas in meeting the child's need for appropriate education and the family's need to keep in close touch.

Some specialities, such as those catering for 'delicate' children, have disappeared altogether. In the past, 'delicate' could cover a range of needs, some very ill-defined. It often provided a useful interim solution for children of families with problems, for those recovering from long illnesses or for those who had been injured and needed both individualized attention and assessment regarding their progress and abilities.

The remaining special schools are becoming places for children with multiple handicap, with severe and very severe disabilities, and generally places for children who are unlikely to be integrated into the usual system at any stage. In turn this has meant that these schools have a greater element of personal caring than teaching, and of teaching very fundamental social skills at the expense of developing learning potentials, and a caretaking as well as an educational function. This has also meant that the ratio of staff to pupils has had to be adjusted and, sometimes due to the lack of available resources, that adjustment has not been easy.

There are many debates about the levels of staff required; what is certain is that it requires people who are committed to the needs of severely handicapped children. It is difficult to attract people of the right calibre who will provide this care, and a lack of career prospects has not added to the solution of the dilemma. Nurses working in special schools are usually full-time, being on-site for all their working hours. Some special schools provide residential care on a weekly basis, some provide residential care on a term basis and others accept the child residentially for unspecified periods. Children in these schools have the same needs as any other child, the needs just multiply and intensify with the handicap. It is of note that those groups who have been most vocal in pressing for integration of all handicapped pupils, are now expressing concern at the nature of the integration which has happened, as well the apparent lack of some provision and support for children with special needs.

Labelling

Another principle underlying the pressure towards integration of children with special needs is to avoid labelling. Attendance at some special schools automatically marked the child as being different, and the label stuck even if the condition improved sufficient to merit 'normal' education. It has been shown that once a child had been identified as being different, the identification persisted even when change occurred, often creating substantial disadvantage (Miller & Gwynne, 1972; Satir, 1978; Featherstone, 1980). Built into any assessment and provision for special needs must be the means of reassessment at regular intervals. Previously it was possible to obtain reassessment on request, but usually the request had to be turned into a firm demand.

The principle of not labelling does appear to have merit, though it causes problems for those who wish to categorize people. In fact, old labels are difficult to overcome, and old-fashioned nomenclature is often heard. The more open-ended approach should prove satisfactory in the long-term, avoiding inaccurate descriptions and simply outlining differences – perhaps school nurses will take as their motto *Vive la difference*.

SUMMARY

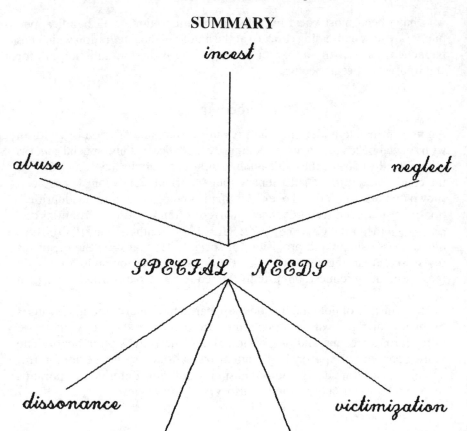

REFERENCES

Brent Borough Council (1986) *A Child in Trust*, report of the enquiry into the circumstances of Jasmine Beckford's death, Brent Council, London.

Featherstone, H. (1980) *A Difference in the Family*, Basic Books, New York.

Kempe, R.S. and Kempe, C.H. (1978) *Child Abuse*, Fontana/Open Books Original, London.

Maslow, A. (1979) *Towards a Psychology of Being*, Reinhold, New York.

Miller, E.J. and Gwynne, G.V. (1972) *A Life Apart*, Tavistock Publication, Tavistock Institute, London (Open University Set Book).

Satir, V. (1978) *Peoplemaking*, Souvenir Press (E & A Ltd), London.

Snowdon Committee Report (1976) *Integrating the Disabled*, National Fund for Research into Crippling Diseases, HMSO, London.

Warnock Committee Report (1978) *Special Educational Needs*, HMSO, London.

5
ROLE AND FUNCTIONS OF SCHOOL NURSES

Currently there is no definitive description of the role and functions of school nurses. Echoes of a role can be found in national legislation relating to the care of schoolchildren, i.e. in the various National Health Service and Education Acts, Statutory Instruments and statements of professional organizations (DHSS, 1977; Health Visitors Association, 1985a and b; Royal College of Nursing, 1974; Society of Area Nurses, 1980). A little more precision is detectable in local government regulations which are concerned mainly with the exclusion and re-entry of pupils with infections or infestations. Some local bye-laws, such as the Inner London Education Authority's (ILEA) regulations governing health and hygiene in schools, come close to role prescription. Government and other reports seek to determine the health care of schoolchildren without clarification of how this is to be accomplished (Scottish Home and Health Department, 1980).

Other chapters in this volume, for example 2, 3 and 9, give closer attention to the implications and applications of some of these reports. Most significant, however, is the Jameson Report (1956), the recommendations of which were accepted, but have not yet – 30 years later – been implemented fully and have never been repealed. This report states that school nurses should be qualified health visitors, and therefore implies that the role and functions are similar, though concentrating on the school-aged section of the population. The functions of the health visitor have not been static during these 30 years; the latest definition and the one on which the health visitor syllabus of education and training is based is reproduced in Appendix A. The concept of 'role progression' will be discussed in Chapter 9, but it is difficult to be clear about this in the context of role diffusion which has occurred through the years.

Far-sighted nurse managers and some medical officers agreed long ago that there was a need to supplement health visiting services and that appropriately trained nurses could effectively provide school health care, in co-operation with health visitors and others. In fact, they perceived the need for a concentrated input by specialized – not specialist – nurses, and that the quality of that input could be enhanced through additional education and training.

JOB DESCRIPTIONS

Reality has led to diversification. In some geographical districts, especially large conurbations, a school nursing service has long and effectively been established. The role and functions of practitioners within these services were defined by localized conditions of service and individual job descriptions. Unfortunately, the latter were and are as varied as employing authorities and often serve to obscure rather than clarify and define. Within job descriptions derived from policies, or because of the lack of defined policy, emphasis is on the obvious, usually physical needs. Hygiene, control of infestation and infection, and assistance at school medical examinations form a large proportion of these descriptions. Within job descriptions based on potential and perceived needs of children, their families and teachers, health teaching, especially on a one-to-one basis, health surveys and health assessments go hand in hand with preventive programmes for control of infections, immunizations and an advisory/supportive function. It needs to be clearly understood that in most instances school nurses, whatever their original qualification, have exceeded the functions inherent in their given job descriptions and that they, together with caring colleagues from other disciplines, are usually in advance of any written document. Their efforts are mainly unsung, undocumented and therefore not officially recognized.

More recently, and especially following the Education Act, 1981, the majority of health authorities, whether in city or county, have considered the health needs of schoolchildren and are endeavouring to establish appropriate care systems with qualified staff. They are faced with constraints such as defective manpower planning, diminishing resources, increasing and changing needs and demands, application of increased knowledge, professional determinants and boundaries. Sadly, it would appear that many of the leaders, i.e. those who established and developed effective school nursing services and came close to defining a role, have been slow in amending their ideas to meet the needs of the present time and are finding difficulties in forward planning.

Prior to the establishment of formal training programmes for school nurses in 1978, the Council for the Education and Training of Health Visitors (CETHV) circulated a description of role and functions on which course content could be based and which was culled from a cross-section of job descriptions. This description was not challenged by the end of the consultation period and, while still not definitive, it proved to be a useful tool. Its omission from later publications was deliberate and significant. It is reproduced as Appendix B.

The Department of Health and Social Security (DHSS) has toyed repeatedly with the idea of providing a nationwide job specification, but to date any drafts are still just that. The only suggestive document to emerge from the Elephant and Castle was the guidance, which never acquired the status of a Circular, on health assessments (DHSS, 1980).

THE ESSENCE OF SCHOOL NURSING

In the absence of a definitive statement it seems appropriate in this context to consider some component parts which form the essence of school nursing, but which are by no means exclusive. Some of these parts are rooted in the history and development of the service and are still a valid aspect of practice, varying in importance with time and context; others are relatively recent additions and a few are essential but not yet fully established.

Being the designated nurse

Since the Education Act 1981 came into effect it has been a requirement that each employing health authority designates a nurse as responsible for co-ordinating the assessment of children with handicap or special educational need. The designated nurse has responsibility to collect and collate reports from nursing colleagues, school nurses, paediatric nurses, staff from accident and emergency departments of hospitals, health visitors or other nurses who may have been involved in the health care of the child under consideration. He/She has to present the case to the multidisciplinary assessment team, support and enhance communications with parents and, in some cases, interpret the final report and recommendations to the parents.

She can advise the provision which may be most appropriate to meet the assessed need, but has to be guided by the team's concensus verdict. The implications of this make her role manifold:

1. She has to be certain that the reports given to her are based on sound professional practice, including use of appropriate assessment tools, up-to-date knowledge and skills, and take account of other known factors such as provision made for siblings, hereditary diseases, progressive illnesses, social conditions and environmental factors affecting decisions, and the understanding and wishes of parents or guardians.
2. She has to be familiar with available resources or their lack, and has to know all channels of referral.
3. She has to be able to communicate at all levels, with colleagues from her own and other disciplines, with policy-makers and with parents and public.
4. She has a responsibility to ensure that reassessment is undertaken at the appropriate time, and that labelling is avoided whenever possible.
5. She may be actively involved in, or advise, formulating care plans and their execution.

Most of those currently designated are Senior Nurses or Nursing Officers with responsibility for other aspects of child health care, such as child abuse and case conferences. Some knowledge of the legal implications of any action or omission is helpful to encompass this part of the role. There is no reason, theoretically speaking, why any school nurse or health visitor should not be designated to this role; the practical difficulties of fulfilling such a role as well as having responsibility for a full case/workload are tremendous.

It has been mentioned that the designated nurse contributes to the assessment of special educational need. It is of note that such assessment can be undertaken upon request by professionals or parents at any time during childhood – from birth to 16 years of age, or 18 years in the case of defined handicap or disease.

Being the named nurse

It has been proved by experience, as well as some evidence, that effective school nursing care can be provided by having a named person responsible for a given population of school-aged children. This enables the nurse as well as the school and service planners to determine case/workloads; allows day-to-day planning of work; gives all parties to the caring process the facility to be aware of the range of activities of the others; highlights the constraints such as time and availability, and adequacy of space or appropriate rooms for carrying out assessment procedures; and clearly demonstrates any gaps in provision.

Many health authorities have instituted the naming of a nurse as carrying responsibility for one or more schools. As yet there are insufficient qualified nurses in post to adjust all workloads to desirable and realistic levels. In all instances the workload must be such as to allow competent professional practice, or the Code of Professional Conduct (UKCC, 1984) is breached in part, with possible consequences for employer and employee.

The named nurse must determine her priorities in caring for the population she serves and liaise with others including managers, teachers and/or therapists in arranging her schedules of work. She will be required to record and report on her activities, i.e. be accountable for her actions, and she must be able to demonstrate how outcomes could be improved or which needs remain unmet. Additionally, she may have to contribute to the training of future colleagues, the professional development of herself and others, interpersonal and interprofessional debate and attend a variety of meetings or sessions.

Subsumed under the description of named nurse are all the variety of responsibilities and tasks which comprise the role and functions in the other ways mentioned in this and other chapters.

Providing school health care and health surveillance

This, of course, is the central feature of any school nurse's role. It sounds so easy, but is fraught with pitfalls. It presumes that the nurse is the expert in health matters, that her knowledge is up-to-date and that she has the skills to practice competently. Health care includes all the other aspects of the role mentioned in this chapter, plus the health teaching of pupils, parents and, wherever necessary, teachers. The last are the experts in teaching but often know very little about health, and even less about disease or handicap and its effects in the classroom or elsewhere.

Health surveillance appears to be the most effective means of providing care for a whole school population. It ensures that each child is seen regularly by the nurse, who can decide whether other actions are required. Children and nurse can establish the sort of relationship which makes contact easy and pleasant, builds trust and confidence and allows the determination of any deviation from the norm before it reaches crisis proportions. Effective health surveillance should be carried out regularly, at least annually. The establishment of a pattern of surveillance is time- and effort-consuming, but it eases the work burden in the long-term. Health surveillance should include, apart from consideration of individuals, identifying patterns of disease or infection in any one setting, recognizing accident high spots and other risk factors, and making appropriate reports and recommendations to overcome these.

Carrying out assessment procedures

Each nurse should be competent to perform a range of assessment procedures, such as hearing and vision testing, weighing and measuring or observation of muscle tone and skeletal posture. The crux and validity of any procedure is that it is performed accurately, and with appropriate instruments which have been correctly maintained, that the professional skill needed to carry it out has been improved beyond basic qualifying level to accommodate most recent applicable research findings, and that results are compared with known and expected norms, leading to formulation of care plans encompassing all these factors.

Assessment is an art and a skill, but it is also a means to an end in that it leads to the early detection of any abnormality giving the chance of treatment and successful outcome. Assessment therefore presupposes efficient referral systems and follow-up, appropriate recording and analysis and professional interpretation of findings. The art of health assessment is using it as a finely honed tool and incidentally and opportunistically for purposes of health teaching.

Advising on health matters

In most instances the school nurse is the only regular visitor to a school with expert knowledge about health matters. That she therefore acts as health adviser to pupils and parents is self-evident. However, she also has a responsibility to advise the headmaster or other authority figure about health hazards particular to that institution or the children within it. She must alert the nurse managers or colleagues in other disciplines, such as medical officers, to hazards which could affect others or the community as a whole and she may be in a position to demonstrate health care deficiencies which affect the population in the immediate or wider environment.

Teachers are responsible for the day-to-day welfare of children in their care, not only educationally but also on a broader basis. Officially the headteacher stands *in loco parentis*, although he usually delegates much of this authority to the contact person, i.e. the classroom teacher. Most teachers are aware of their responsibilities and those aspects which may be outwith their competence. Increasingly, teachers seek professional help and support to fulfil their role effectively. They are concerned with the implications of integrating handicapped pupils into 'normal', which often means difficult, settings. They are worried about the handling or side-effects of prescribed medications, of children who may miss lessons by attendance at treatment or therapy, of the effects on other children when an individual is unwell in class or functionally different. They may wish to adapt the classroom environment to suit the pupils within it, but find this difficult or impossible and greatly benefit by advice and reassurance.

On many occasions teachers are concerned with aspects of their own health, ability to overcome stress and generally seek ways to enhance their abilities to cope. They therefore welcome the opportunity to discuss these issues, to feel supported and often to be advised on how to reach appropriate channels of professional help. The nurse has to use listening skills as well as advising, and be aware of the limits of her expertise and role as a referral agent. Nurses are generally perceived as being knowledgeable, sympathetic and available, whereas doctors are seen as useful in dealing with major crises, but not so approachable or useful as confidantes. The stresses engendered by recent changes and events in the education sector have increased substantially the demands made on nurses by teachers.

Being involved with immunizations

School nurses will be involved in carrying out immunization and vaccination programmes. Their main function is to explain the reasons for each type of procedure, to verify that courses of injections are completed at the right time and to follow up defaulters. They may be involved in the collection and collation of data which leads to determination of the state of resistance to certain diseases within the population.

In some health districts it may be the policy for nurses to carry the function of administering immunizations. In these instances assurances have to be sought that the nurse has the appropriate training, skill and knowledge to carry out the procedure, to recognize contraindications, deal with adverse reactions and have immediate access for referral of serious or doubtful instances. The district policy should be clearly stated, preferably in writing. Subscription to, or deviance from, nationally recommended patterns should be acknowledged openly, and such matters as indemnity insurance cover and other legalities completed. In most instances the responsibility for correct administration of immunization and vaccination agents is vested in the school medical officer or general medical practitioner. If this is the case, the school nurse may have a delegated function for carrying out the procedure; aspects of accountability and responsibility should be negotiated and clarified before action.

In any event, school nurses must be familiar with the possible side-effects of immune substances, the contraindications for administration, correct dosages, and correct storage and preparation for use. They have to be aware of emergency treatments required in cases of anti-reaction and report any sign of persistent reaction to any batch of materials used.

Policy regarding the timings of immunizations change with advances in science and medicine or related new knowledge, and nurses have to be aware of the changes and the reasons for them. Nurses also have to keep abreast of public debate about issues relating to immunizations and be able to state *known* facts, without succumbing to personal bias.

An important facet of the nurse's role is the obtaining of consent for any procedure to be carried out. Consent should be given in full knowledge of all the facts, by parents or guardian and the young person. 'Informed consent' is a legal conundrum with a range of implications, not all of which are very clear. In this country actions appear to be based on assumptions that professional practitioners, including nurses and doctors, know what they are doing, and the public or recipient is sufficiently informed to make on-the-spot decisions; in practice that may mean signing a form. These assumptions are rarely challenged, usually only when something misfires. The notion of 'informed consent' has been very hotly and publicly debated in the United States where the information-giving and understanding of information processes have been successfully challenged in the law-courts.

Carrying out screening procedures

It appears to be generally accepted that screening procedures form part of child assessment or health surveillance, though screening procedures can be totally divorced from any other facet of health care and may exceed those commonly used by nurses or doctors. Screening procedures can be developed for many things and, in terms of health care, for all age-groups.

The usual range of screening procedures used are based on a few major assumptions and interpretations of results. The execution of the procedure and recording of data should reflect this. Some of these assumptions are:

1. Screening is part of primary prevention, and should cover a total given population. It seeks to detect faults or malfunction sufficiently early to prevent deterioration or to enable cure.
2. Screening, as part of secondary prevention, addresses a known 'evil' and, by processes of detection and subsequent elimination reduces risks – head infestations and some infectious diseases come into this category.
3. Screening means that treatment and referral for such treatment is

available, and that time-lapse between detection, through screening and action, by treatment, is minimal.
4. The person carrying out the screening procedure is competent and adequately trained to do so.
5. The results of screening are known to be cost-effective in humane, human and fiscal terms.
6. Anxiety is lessened by the screening procedure, not engendered or increased by it.

It can be seen that some of the assumptions are perhaps more realistic than others, and that the obverse could be true in each instance. The implications for school nursing and school health are manifold, not least to ensure that procedures are used which meet, for the most part, the positive side of these statements and that those who carry out screening procedures are able to communicate what they are doing on many levels, and explain, elucidate, and reassure.

Preventing illness, deterioration or the spread of infection

Health surveillance and screening procedures are tools of primary prevention, covering a whole range of situations. It is important that in situations such as schools the spread of infection is avoided as much as possible. School nurses may have to advise about incubation periods of diseases, of the length of time of exclusion from school or other contact with peers. Occasionally, they may have to sound the alert to danger zones within schools, such as ponds which are rarely cleaned, or cafeteria areas where the debris is inadequately removed.

Periodically, the old infectious diseases make reappearances, some remain with us, and fewer people are able to recognize and differentiate between signs and symptoms. Nurses, especially if they happen to have personal contact with children in family life, are more likely than doctors to have seen and dealt with diseases which are troublesome, but not particularly dangerous, such as scarlatina. Newer diseases, or old diseases new to the Western World, may be imported through travel. The most common reminders of school holidays abroad are gastric upsets of various origins and severity. Methods of disinfection of commonly used facilities, such as toilets, may have to be advised – though the days when school nurses went round with carbolic soap and disinfectant are hopefully past.

Having an occupational health input

Since schools and colleges have been included in the provision of the Health and Safety at Work etc. Act 1974, and although schools apparently form the 'etc.' the school nurse's function which relates to safety has been officially recognized. In most instances she is not responsible directly for applying safety standards, but she may be able to pinpoint danger spots, alert head-teachers and inform teachers about the correct use and storage of dangerous materials, ensure that fire precautions are adhered to, for example that desks and books are not blocking emergency exits, and highlight areas where accidents are too frequent. She could be instrumental in arranging instruction about safety aspects, such as road and home safety. More directly, she could help to ensure that safety clothing, goggles or headgear are worn and that such clothing is available.

Unless the school nurse is permanently based in a school she cannot carry out first-aid, but she should verify that each school has trained first-aiders on site at all times. She may be involved, though not exclusively, in their initial and subsequent training. Even when a school nurse is permanently on site, the first-aid function should be carefully negotiated, since her broader remit may mitigate against provision of first-aid. Despite being a nurse, her knowledge and skills in emergency treatments may be rusty. Many authorities require recent completion of either a Red Cross or St. John's Ambulance course of all those designated as first-aiders.

Being a referral agent

Some aspects of the nurse's work will result in requiring the services of other experts on behalf of the child, such as opticians, speech therapists, doctors or social workers. The skills and arts required in being a referral agent include effective communication, knowledge of available resources, realistic use of these resources and some persistence as well as tact and diplomacy. The most desirable referral is a direct, person-to-person one with feedback of outcomes; however, this is not always possible. Feedback and follow-up are concomitants of referral.

Referral is accomplished most speedily when written communications are preceded by verbal contact. This should be the norm in referral to colleagues, such as from school nurse to health visitor or nursing officer or vice versa. It is also possible in contacts with other caring agencies, including social workers and doctors, but is desirable and helpful in most instances. Referral implies the consent of the referred, and yet again raises the issue of informed consent. Occasionally, decisions will have to be made about referring a person, especially a child, without permission or consent. These decisions are especially crucial in instances or suspicions of abuse, neglect or some contagious diseases. They may also be relevant when there is evidence or suspicion of drug or solvent abuse, bullying or severe discrimination.

Reporting matters of concern or importance

Reports may be verbal or written, requested or self-initiated. In any event they form part of school nursing practice. They should be clearly written, differentiating between data gained through screening and assessment procedures, and professional opinion based on the interpretation of the data. Professional opinion and judgement are valuable, provided that the base for them is sound and reliable and that the rationale for the opinion and judgement are clearly stated. Information received from others, colleagues, teachers, parents or neighbours and friends may need to be recorded and reported, but should be clearly identified as information received, and to what extent it has been possible to substantiate this information.

Reports may be required for a variety of reasons and addressed to different recipients. They should be worded in such a way that they can be understood clearly by the addressee, avoiding jargon, and giving indication about possible lines of action, or the consequences if action is not taken. All documents should be dated, identifiable regarding their origin and request a place and deadline for response. The last is specially important if the report results in inaction, or if a decision is made not to act. Written records of this decision could assist materially in future judgements. The range and reasons for reports are wide, and the following examples are not exclusive. Some reports may be most effective if they follow a given format; others should be based on the exigencies of the situation.

The head-teacher may need information about the health status of a pupil in order to achieve appropriate tuition and care; the nurse may wish to draw the head-teacher's attention to a matter of general concern or safety, or report concern about an individual; the designated nurse may require an assessment or screening report to incorporate in the formal multidisciplinary assessment procedure; nurse management may need or request to be informed about the outcomes of special programmes, innovations, teaching activities, notable and notifiable disease or handicap patterns or be alerted to shortfalls in provision, including staffing and availability and maintenance of equipment. Any professional person, such as a school nurse, may feel it is important that proposals are made at local and national levels about aspects of professional practice or standards.

Reporting about individual children can pose a dilemma for the reporter. Professional concern may indicate that a situation is noted for further action by the nurse and/or others; personal concern may wish to safeguard the confidence reposed in the nurse by the child or its parents. There are as many answers to this dilemma as there are possible situations, and decisions can only be made in the full knowledge of all factors. When professional concerns or child protection outweigh concerns about confidentiality, the child and/or its parents or guardian may have to be informed that the matter cannot any longer be kept confidential. This may make interpersonal relationships difficult, but an honest, open approach usually has better results than secrecy and deviousness and enables relationships to be re-established on a secure footing.

An additional dilemma is confidentiality of and access to reports. Some reports are confidential documents between professionals and caring agencies, and copies are usually filed in records. In the majority of instances when confidentiality of written materials is claimed, this is a misnomer, as a range of people will be able to gain access if they so desire. I would like to suggest that, except in the case of discussion between two people which is not mentioned to a third party, confidentiality is a myth. It is therefore preferable to make reports accessible to all those concerned, and to ensure that the nature of the document is not open to misinterpretation.

Within the guidance to the implementation to the Education Act 1981, parental access to summaries of assessment reports and recommendations is assured. Parents and other adults can gain legal access to most records pertaining to the children in their care; it is preferable to move to a system of limited, open access than to be involved in legal wrangles. The matter is dealt with, though sketchily, in the Data Protection Act 1985 and currently a Bill is in the process of becoming law which will allow access to personal records, including medical and school ones, to the individual affected by the record – in the case of children that would extend to their parents or guardian.

Recording information

Record-keeping is the bane of all professional practice. It is time-consuming and often appears to be a waste of effort. However, accurate recording is essential if service provision is to be efficient, effective and appropriate. The purposes of recording are manifold, a few are selected here for consideration:

1. Records should demonstrate professional practice, its extent and value. They delineate the achievement of objectives and the adaptation of plans to meet new or changed needs and circumstances.
2. Records are one means of assessing competence, of monitoring service provision and developments.

3. Records are tools. In the case of child assessment, they should clearly demonstrate developmental progress, and whether the progression is within the range of 'normal'. The type of record used for this purpose may vary, as it does for any purpose, but percentile charts are one useful and cheap means which have proved themself through many vicissitudes. Where progress is not noted, where there is regression rather than progresion, or where there is substantive deviation from accepted norms, records should form the basis for referral and action.

4. They should facilitate the determination of patterns of health and disease for a given population or geographical area, and allow forward planning to meet health needs, preventive measures to be taken and health promotion activities to be targetted. Where there is a sudden or gradual change in patterns this can provide a timely indicator of a potential problem.

5. The use of records as a teaching tool is highly effective. It can lead to the development of care plans between child, parent, nurse and others and implicit or explicit agreement to follow such plans to successful conclusions.

The storage of records has always been a problem. They are rarely the right size for any file, cupboard or holder, nor is there facility to have them at the most convenient site for use and access. This may now ease with the advent of computerized recording systems, but these require the acquisition of the new skills by health care professionals. The suggestion, made in many ways and by many groups and people, that individuals should be responsible for holding their own records therefore merits consideration. This may also solve the dilemmas of confidentiality. Experimental schemes, e.g. in Portsmouth and Southampton health districts, have proved successful (Health Visitor, 1985).

Confidentiality of records, as well as that of reports, has long been an issue for debate. The current confused situation is that the record itself is the property of the health authority, which is responsible for its retention until seven years after it ceases to be used. At the same time the information on the record is the property of the child or its parents, with responsibility for its accuracy vested in the recorder of the information or data. There are great similarities between records and reports in that authorities and professional groups are reluctant to grant parental rights of access. 'Open recording' is being advocated widely and appears greatly preferable to producing information on demand or under duress.

Records can also be part of evidence if legal issues or challenges occur. This fact has created greater consciousness of the need for accuracy and avoidance of time-lapse in maintaining the record.

The principles underlying recording are the same whether the system is manual or technological. The replacing of manual systems by machines is likely to increase rapidly, following the implementation in 1987 of the Koerner Report's recommendations to have 'data sets' for national and local accountability (Steering Group on Health Services Information, 1983). Statisticians, pressure groups and official bodies such as community health councils (CHCs) are likely to request data at frequent intervals. The increasing availability and decreasing cost of computers is accelerating the rate of change.

Health teaching

Each school nurse is automatically a health teacher, whether she participates in formal groups or simply explains what she is doing at a particular time. The skills and arts of teaching can be refined and developed to meet the range of situations in which teaching can take place. Not all school nurses wish to be part of formal teaching schedules; most, however, will be prepared to advise on content and materials which could and should be used for particular topics, or on experts available to help the teacher cover health-related subjects. Formal teaching is not the nurse's prime function, but many are happy and very capable to be part of the curriculum in their named schools. Health teaching can only be effective if it is a part of a planned, continuous process; *ad hoc* sessions may occasionally be necessary but are rarely productive.

Subject matter can be varied, but must be adapted to suit the age-group, demonstrate awareness of individual needs and cultural mores and differences. When teaching, it is of paramount importance that the subject matter is based on the best available information or research findings, and practical changes such as those resulting from application of technology to medicine should be reflected.

As in report-writing and record-keeping, the means and methods of communication are vital ingredients. Teaching requires language skills, supported by skills in using supplementary materials. The language must be one that can be understood unequivocally by the pupils, though it should also reflect the professionalism of the presenter. More about this dilemma will be presented in Chapter 11.

Nurses may be requested to participate in campaigns or large-scale programmes addressing specific health issues. Whatever form participation takes, it is important that the outcomes are evaluated and used to benefit future planning and nursing input.

Developing care plans

Pressures to provide efficient and effective services has led to acceptance that a process approach is a useful method or tool for developing care plans, and acting upon them. Most experienced nurses have used this approach for a long time, but it has rarely been formalized. There have also been weaknesses in evaluating and reviewing, or at least there has been little evidence that these stages of any plan were completed. In view of what has already been stated about reporting and recording and the requirements of accountability, formalizing the methodology seems relevant and appropriate. The establishment of the means requires thought and time, though it should save time and trouble in the longer term. Care plans may be based on 'the nursing process', though this is only the application of a more general concept to nursing. The stages of any plan or process should be:

1. Collecting data and information, including availability of resources.
2. Interpreting the above and formulating a plan.
3. Acting on the plan.
4. Evaluating actions and outcomes.
5. Reviewing and revising the plan, supplementing data.
6. Acting on the new plan (Figure 5.1).

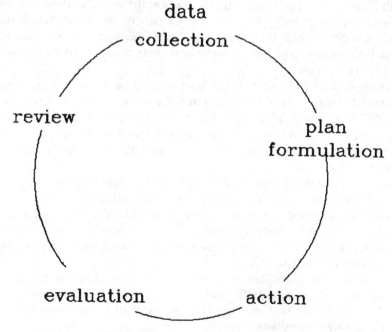

Figure 5.1   Stages in a care plan

Any recording system involving this type of activity should be concise, clear, and understandable to all involved at any stage, but not of extravagant length.

The formulation of care plans can be beneficial to school nursing practice. It is already inherent in good practice. The material for the initial stage is available through initial assessments; the second phase is a means of consultation with others; the third phase involves child, parents and others as much as the nurse; the fourth phase is exciting and can improve practice; and the last phase represents continuance and follow-through. All phases are, of course, inherently repetitive, with greater emphasis on the last ones for any one, like a school nurse, who has to plan health promotion, disease prevention, rehabilitation or protection in the medium- and long-term, rather than cure, which should be immediate or short-term. A well-formulated care plan should be an aid to communication and memory as well as fulfilling its primary purpose.

Participating in creating a healthy environment

School health care is essential to enable the child to achieve his learning potential without additional risks. The importance of personal health is obvious, as persistent or recurrent illness leads to under-achievement in school. However, there comes a point when the best health care will be ineffective because the child's circumstances mitigate against well-being. The nurse may feel powerless to effect changes which would lead to improvement. Each nurse has to decide when, where and how it is appropriate to mobilize other resources; for example, stimulating civic action, campaigning for lead-free petrol or the reduction of noise levels. Many of these issues are ethical, philosophical or political – nurses of the 1980s and 1990s cannot remain unaware of the pressures put upon them and their clientele and the powers and pressures they can use in return.

On a practical level, nurses have to involve themselves with ensuring that the immediate environment is as hygienic and hazard-free as possible. A healthy environment, apart from hazards in eating, playing areas and toilets, may include action about litter on access roads, unmanned crossings close to schools, or reporting suspected kerb-crawlers and drug-pushers. It means being aware of what other organizations are doing or might usefully be doing and how to stimulate activities that provide desirable and welcome support.

Serving as a member of several teams

Team membership is never easy, it requires constant effort and adjustment of functions, relationships and ideas. Effective team membership implies trust in each other, respect for others' professional roles and boundaries, sharing of information and knowledge, as well as providing and taking constructive criticism. The benefits of team membership far outweigh the disadvantages – it should lead to improved services to client groups and individuals, facilitate personal and professional growth and increase job satisfaction. Team membership implies *equality* in every sense of that word.

School nurses are in the invidious position of being members of several teams, sometimes at the same time. The educational team may accord full, partial or temporary membership; the nursing team in the community is the obvious metier, the primary health care team is the desirable goal. Additionally, and at times, the school nurse may be a member of an assessment team or of a team of specialists. The range of implied activities could be confusing and formidable, each individual has to prioritize her contribution, and thereby membership status, in any given situation. Each team is a dynamic organism with constantly changing parameters, and while at any one time the nurse's position may be peripheral, at another time she may be the team leader.

Being accountable

Nurses have always been accountable, in fact accountability is implicit in any form of professional practice. In recent years demands for accountability have become more public. There has to be accountability at all levels of the profession, from the senior manager to the most junior probationer. The forms this process takes are many and varied, and can be very formalized or very flexible. Acceptance of the system current within the employing authority is part of the usual conditions of service for an employee.

Accountability has much wider implications and the nature of the real thing compared with expediency should be carefully considered. First and foremost, any professional person is accountable for her actions to herself. Part of good professional practice is knowledge of self, limitations, prejudices and how to overcome the last. Stringent accountability to self will lead to confidence when facing managerial or public scrutiny. Some professional groups, such as general medical practitioners, are moving towards systems of self-audit; whether such formalization is essential for good practice is open to debate. It is evident, however, that each person needs to examine her performance at regular intervals, to ensure that competencies remain more than adequate, that knowledge remains up-to-date and that skills have improved, not suffered, through overuse.

Second, each practitioner is accountable to colleagues and peers. If there is any shortfall in practice, the load on colleagues is increased; this is generally undesirable but becomes unwarrantable in times of constraint or lack of resources. Nursing, like any other professional group, has always contained some members who have performed less well than others. Colleagues have usually been too kind and caring to remark on this or take any action. During times of distress or crisis, the collegiate relationship should lead to help and support, but beyond this any cover-up becomes questionable. In the relative isolation of any work within community settings, it is easy to malfunction without being noticed and both the support system and the peer audit may fail. It may not be pertinent to establish formal systems of peer audit, but informal systems should be made to function effectively.

Third, each school nurse, as well as any other practitioner, is accountable to the client, in this case child and parent. The client has the right to expect a competent, knowledgeable and efficient service carried out with the minimum of disturbance. Within this, the client has the right to expect full explanations of any actions, the right to consultation about proposals relating to personal health, and preservation of privacy. Until recently, clients have held nurses in high esteem and rarely questioned their pronouncements or actions; the present well- or even mis-informed, educated public means that challenges are more frequent. The client usually requests verbal accountability, but may in future demand a written statement about any matter.

Next, the nurse is accountable to her employer. The employer is, in turn, accountable for the use of resources, including manpower, and has a monitoring role in seeing that the service is provided correctly and as effectively as possible. Last, but not least, accountability may take a public format, through local or national organizations, press and other forms of mass media, correspondence and participation in community activities.

The public, being the taxpayers/paymasters and the recipients of care, have a right to be fully involved. Professional secrecy and mysteriousness are no longer acceptable. Table 5.2 shows the various and complex channels of accountability.

Having professional responsibility

All of these points imply professional responsibility to clients, colleagues, employers and public (Baly, 1975). Additionally, there is the responsibility to contribute to professional standing and development. On a personal level this means acknowledging strengths and weaknesses, sharing the former and taking action to overcome the latter. Continuing education is a shared responsibility between practitioner and employer: for the first as overt recognition that nothing remains static, including knowledge and skills; for

Table 5.1 Accountability

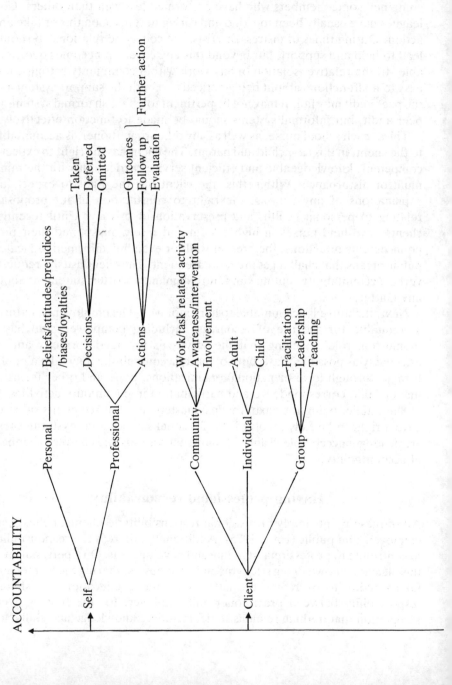

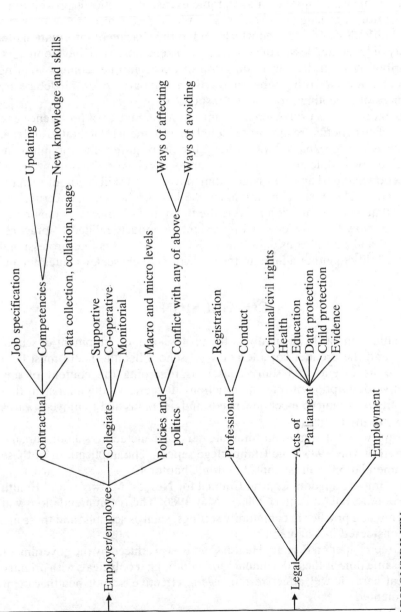

Job specification
Updating
Competencies
New knowledge and skills
Data collection, collation, usage

Supportive
Co-operative
Monitorial

Macro and micro levels
Ways of affecting
Conflict with any of above
Ways of avoiding

Registration

Conduct

Criminal/civil rights
Health
Education
Data protection
Child protection
Evidence

Contractual

Collegiate

Policies and politics

Professional

Acts of Parliament

Employment

Employer/employee

Legal

RESPONSIBILITY

the second as a safeguard for competent practice. The simplest form of professional updating is the perusal of journals. Those available cover a wide range of topics. Time, or its lack, is the usual excuse for sketchy reading; this would not be an acceptable excuse if practice is proven to be deficient or knowledge inadequate with ready access to relevant information. Methods can be devised which lead to the sharing of information at a variety of levels and lessen the time taken to keep abreast of developments. Contributing to professional education of peers and newcomers, sharing research findings, writing papers and articles and participating in debate are instances of accepting professional responsibility.

Membership of a professional organization is a matter of preference and choice. The benefits are that professional development is facilitated and that new ideas can be explored with others. It does require some commitment, though a few people are 'sleeping' members, relying on the organizations' protection and perhaps their negotiating powers and skills without reciprocal activity. These 'sleepers' minimize the benefits which can accrue, and forget that any organization reflects the input and calibre of its members.

Nurses now have a Code of Professional Conduct, related to practice, practical and ethical considerations (UKCC, 1984). It is one professional responsibility to either adhere to this code or actively seek its amendment.

CONCLUSION

Diversification has been an ally to the professional development of school nurses and the broader considerations of school health. There must be a limit to its extent, and some consensus regarding the content of any definitive description of role and functions. It seems vitally important that flexibility is in-built to meet new needs and demands and to move towards the twenty-first century.

A review of all community nursing services, including school nursing, reported in May 1986 – the Cumberlege report. The implications of these recommendations will be considered in Chapter 12.

The United Kingdom Central Council for Nurses, Midwives and Health Visitors reported on Project 2000 in May 1986. The recommendations will affect nursing practice in community settings, such as schools, and these are also considered in Chapter 12.

A Green Paper on Primary Health Care was produced by the government at the same time as these documents and, although it only deals with primary medical care, it will affect resources for effective school health care if implemented.

Parallel with the three major documents, a committee has been formed to consider the role and function of medical officers in the public health system. The outcome is not known, but the effect may be significant, especially for the role and functions of the school nurse.

Professional organizations, such as the Health Visitors Association (HVA) and the Amalgamated School Nurses Association (ASNA), have recently established working groups to consider the role, functions and professional development of school nurses. It is not yet known when they will report or how their reports will affect practice, nor how their findings will fit into the proposals contained in the other documents.

SUMMARY

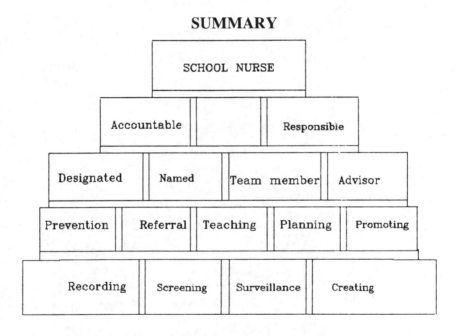

REFERENCES

Baly, M. (1975) *Professional Responsibility*, H.M. & M., Aylesbury.

DHSS (1977) *Nursing in Primary Health Care*, CNO(77)8, DHSS, London

DHSS (1980) 'Suggested programme of child health surveillance'. Supplement to *Good Practice in Prevention*, HC(78)5 (1978), DHSS, London.

Health Visitor (1985) Parents held record cards, *Journal of the Health Visitors Association*, London.

HVA (1985a) *Health Visiting and School Nursing – The Future*, HVA, London.

HVA (1985b) Memorandum to the Review Body for Nursing Staff, Midwives, Health Visitors and Professions Allied to Medicine, Section VII and Appendix 3, HVA, London.

Jameson Committee Report (1956) *Enquiry into Health Visiting*, HMSO, London.

Royal College of Nursing (1974) *Role of the School Nurse*, RCN, London.

Scottish Home and Health Department (1980) *Towards Better Health Care for School Children in Scotland*, HMSO, Edinburgh.

Society of Area Nurses – Child Health (1980) *Review of the School Nursing Service*

Steering Group on Health Services Information (1983–85) *Collection of Information about Services for and in the Community*, chairman Mrs E. Koerner, 5th report, Part I, Chapts. 3, 4 and 5. HMSO, London.

UKCC (1984) *Code of Professional Conduct for Nurses, Midwives and Health Visitors*, UKCC, London.

6
TOOLS FOR THE TRADE

It is obvious that competent practice requires suitable tools and equipment to ensure successful outcomes. It is also obvious, when visiting schools and talking with school nurses, that some of these tools go unrecognized, others are undervalued and some are conspicuous by their absence. At one time there was some excuse, though of doubtful validity, for inadequate provision. This time has passed and it is the responsibility of each nurse, together with the manager to whom she is accountable, to ensure that competent practice is made possible, and that fundamental competencies can be enhanced by improved provision. It is appreciated that improvement of provision often requires commitment of resources. Most of the tools needed by nurses are not very costly. The benefits, such as saving time through avoiding make-shift materials and the need for repetition and accuracy on which decisions can be based, far outweigh the cost. The following tools have been selected as being basic to practice; the number could and should be increased to accommodate innovations and technical as well as scientific developments.

KNOWLEDGE

Each nurse requires base-line knowledge, which should be acquired through professional training and updating. The knowledge base is constantly shifting, and no practitioner can depend on the information gleaned during initial training courses. In fact, it is debatable how much, and equally how much relevant, knowledge is retained from any initial training programme and how long this retention lasts. It seems a matter of major importance, therefore, that each nurse not only becomes aware of possible gaps in her own knowledge base, but institutes a system of access to references and information to aid recall. It is better to defer a decision or action for a short period until information and knowledge can be verified, than to make the wrong decision through ignorance.

The value and importance of reading current literature has been mentioned in Chapter 5. It would be a difficult, if not impossible, task to be aware of the detail of all new materials, plans and proposals. Systems must therefore be devised to overcome possible shortfalls. One way is for each colleague to take responsibility for scanning an agreed range of journals and books and alerting others to articles and chapters of relevance. Another means is for senior or specialist staff to shoulder this responsibility and become responsible for the dissemination of information. A mixture of both may be the most successful, but neither absolves individual responsibility.

The lasting value of initial education and training has been questioned; it is therefore important to establish systems whereby retention of learning is enhanced, and whereby learning of special importance to the particular post is ensured. Post-registration courses, such as the course in school nursing, are therefore part of the answer. Few post-registration courses are a mandatory requirement for practice; in fact, mandate has been shown to inhibit progress. Employers who wish to ensure that service requirements are met, will also ensure that their staff is appropriately qualified to fulfil the roles and is able to act without constant supervision or guidance, i.e. that all staff have had the relevant preparation for the job. Employees who continue to function without the relevant background and without arguing the case for post-registration training may also be deemed to be at fault.

Refresher courses

A few nursing disciplines, such as midwifery, have always had the opportunity and requirement for regular updating refresher courses. Others have had variable opportunity, some have not had any and, regrettably, a few have had this opportunity and have not utilized it. Most health authorities are now establishing, or have established, programmes of in-service updating courses; many authorities will consider requests for attendance at such courses, which have to be prioritized to match available resources. The most successful method of updating by course attendance will be when the need for a specific course, which ironically may be a generalized refresher course, has been identified and agreed between nurse and manager, and the most suitable venue, time and content negotiated. The principle of regular updating for all nursing staff has been established by the four National Boards of Nursing, Midwifery and Health Visiting and UKCC. The completion of a live register, due in 1987, with periodic registration for all, is the first step towards formalizing this requirement. At a yet unspecified date continued registration will become dependent on proof of updated knowledge and competence.

Each person who has attended a course or conference can and should contribute to the updating of others in the health care teams or the staff of the district. This can be achieved by reporting back, describing what has been gained and circulating documents which have been newly acquired. This is one way of sharing knowledge with others and learning from each other. Generally, sharing information with people from nursing and other disciplines can enhance the base-lines of all those involved. Sometimes considerable effort has to be made to ensure that sharing of knowledge is facilitated. Multi-professional meetings and discussion groups, or lunch clubs, are another step in the direction of maintaining and enhancing knowledge.

A great deal of knowledge is gained through experience. The competence acquired by this means cannot be negated, though it is important to check the experience for relevance against other facts and information. Each person has different perceptions of experience gained, and there are many arguments about the pertinence of depth versus breadth. Both appear to be important at different times and for different reasons. Experience should be used to enhance practice, but this can only be beneficial if the first is analysed, and peculiarities acknowledged.

Knowledge forms the basis for professional judgement. Some people claim that they act instinctively or intuitively. I would like to suggest that professional intuition is based on unanalysed experience and unrecognized knowledge and skill. It should therefore be possible to substantiate instinct and intuition.

SKILLS

Many of the skills required of a nurse are inherent in the job description and acquired through both training and experience. The practical skills are those of assessment and screening, of prophylactic measures and treatments, of recognition of disease and difficulty and of providing any care that involves a recognizable procedure.

Equally important, or often more so, are the skills which are intangible and more difficult to delineate and define. The most important of all are the range of communication skills. It was considered sufficient at one time that a nurse used her social skills for communicating, and that the constant contact with people from all social and age-groups would endow her with the ability to communicate effectively. This has been proved wrong. All the evidence appears to show that effective communication can occur only when inherent talents have been developed, when conscious effort has been made to improve upon it, and when different forms of communications have been learned, together with understanding of the two-, or more, way nature of the process. Currently, much work and research is being undertaken to establish a successful base-line for communications in nursing; the published work of Ashworth (1980), Argyle (1982) and Kagan (1985) are but a selection from a rapidly expanding field.

Writing skills

Written communications are essential for record-keeping and report-writing. It is a sad reflection that many nurses continue to have difficulties in expressing themselves on paper, and that their otherwise valuable statements are often ignored because they are either illegible or ill-formulated.

An essential of written communication is to present data in a logical sequence, to extract the points which are most pertinent, and to draw conclusions or make recommendations in a form which is clear and understandable to the recipient. A subsidiary to a clearly and succinctly written communication is to be aware of whom to address it, to choose the most suitable time, and to request a response. The latter is often most effective if a deadline or date is given, so that follow-up, which is often essential, can occur. An extension and utilization of skills in written communication is to contribute to professional journals, or to produce papers for debate and discussion. In recent years British nurses have developed considerably in this direction, they still have not caught up with their American counterparts.

Verbal communications

Verbal communication skills are the bread and butter of all nurses, but vitally important when considering health education, health promotion and disease prevention, all of which form a part of the school nurse's role. Effective verbal communication requires the facility to establish dialogue at all levels, with people from many different backgrounds and of all ages. It requires a presentation of self, which indicates an understanding of others' expressions of thoughts and feelings, and a vocabulary which can accommodate dialects, accents or limited use of English. The vocabulary used by the professional must be neither full of incomprehensible jargon, nor so simplified that it appears patronizing. Accents, if they are genuine, do not appear to matter, but affectations do grate on many client groups. Children are especially quick to detect any sham or prevarication, and will be reluctant to establish the necessary trust.

Language usage changes, sometimes very rapidly, and while it is not generally essential to alter one's own approach, one has to be very aware of changed or double meanings of words. The most used verbal communication is, of course, in the one-to-one situation. However, the telephone, tape-recorder and video or television have all become normal means of communication. Each requires the use of this skill in a different way. The first two are especially important as other clues, such as nonverbal signals, are absent. With experience, it becomes very easy to detect signals like anger and frustration in the speaker even if attempts are made to cover them.

Verbal facility is used to chat, discuss, instruct, order or as an expression of opinion. Each category depends not only on the words used, but also on the inflexions and the perceived status of the communicator. It is very important that verbal signals are received and understood in the way they are intended. Much miscommunication and serious misunderstanding occurs because it is assumed that the same meaning is given to words by the parties involved in the communication. Often it has been shown that something completely different was received than intended, and that this can be a barrier to effective actions and outcomes. Questions are one means of ensuring understanding; allowing space or time to assimilate verbal messages and formulate responses are more effective ones. If verbal communication forms the basis for teaching or learning, reinforcement has to be built in. Sometimes there is miscommunication because too much information is presented in one mass; in such a case the component parts may need to be determined and reiterated.

Some communicators, nurses included, have habits which can irritate. The unfortunate thing about these habits is that the person is usually unaware of them, or that one habit is replaced by another, for example, continually saying 'you know', 'd'you see', 'well'.

Nonverbal communication

Nonverbal communications complement verbal ones, and on occasion replace them. The complement occurs when gestures or posture give out

Nursing in educational settings

messages which indicate interest, attention and care. Dissonance occurs when gestures or grimaces contradict the words spoken. Many people react first to nonverbal clues, and either they will allow effective information exchange or they form a barrier. This is especially crucial when attempting to communicate with a person from a different social or cultural background; it is too easy for both sides to talk *at* each other not *with* each other. Where a known language barrier exists, the effort at communication is usually overt, and attempts are made to find a formula for understanding. When there is no apparent language barrier the situation can deteriorate to farcical levels. The language of touch, smile, eye contact, grimace or posture should not be underestimated; it may need to be adapted to become significant at the interface between classes and cultures.

One very vital component of communication skills is *listening*. It sounds so easy; we all claim we listen more than we talk. However, many people only half-listen, while some hear what they wish to hear and ignore the remainder, and some do not listen at all. This does not apply to someone who is actually hard of hearing, because usually this person will make every effort to listen, whether with their ears, with help of hearing aids or by lip-reading. People within the range of normal hearing are bombarded by sounds and often 'switch off'; they select their input. During professional practice such selection can be deleterious and dangerous. Listening skills allow the other person to collect their thoughts, express their feelings and concerns, however inadequately, and appreciate tones and pauses which may provide significant leads to unexpressed concerns.

Listening skills will include hearing the nuances of the spoken word, not interpreted in the listener's terms, but interpreted in the light of knowledge and understanding of the speaker. Effective listening can create a climate for discussion of the most banal or the most delicate matters, of sympathy and understanding and of paving the way for realistic, acceptable advice. It should be supportive, and often allows the speaker to sort his/her own information and understanding or gaps in this, and to formulate solutions to problems. Good listening is not intrusive, does not breach privacy and creates trust. It is a skill; it can be developed into an art. It takes a lot of practice, patience and a high degree of professionalism.

Communications form the essence of interpersonal skills, a requirement for any one, like a school nurse, who has to work with people, within teams and who has to negotiate between agencies and individuals. Several books have been written about interpersonal skills; those by Kagan *et al.* (1986), and Satir (1978) are representative of this group with self-help manuals to allow professional development, from a collaborative venture between training institutions (Barnet and Manchester Colleges, 1986).

ATTITUDES

Attitudes, including biases and prejudices, influence practice and can affect understanding and the interpretation of information or new knowledge. They are often gained subconsciously, insidiously and accepted as part of the individual. Any professional person needs to examine her attitudes – to people, to work, to issues and to a range of situations. This examination does not have to occur in public; it is a personal matter, and should result in either amending those attitudes which are detrimental to professional practice, or an acceptance and conscious acknowledgement. Those attitudes which affect practice may become the subject of public or management scrutiny, affecting in turn the selection for posts, courses and career development. There are formal measuring devices, such as personality tests, which seek to determine attitudes. Some have proved helpful in selection or management terms, but none have been proved to be conclusive. Attitude change is not easy; it requires determination and effort, and often has to be repeated throughout life and career. Open mindedness and receptivity to ideas and new knowledge are vital stages in attitude formation and change.

The attitudes of each professional person may coincide or conflict with those of their client group. It is therefore equally important to be aware of the attitudes held by those whom one attempts to serve, and to accept and accommodate them.

Of the vast range of attitudes which make up a person and their life, three appear to be of paramount importance to school nurses:

1. Honesty in approach, leading to open and fair dealing with any situation and facilitating partnership, reciprocity and acceptance.
2. Tolerance, allowing others the freedom and opportunity to express their beliefs and act according to their tenets. Tolerance does not mean any lowering of one's own standards, but it allows influence on equal terms. Children are among the most intolerant of creatures; in fact, it takes considerable maturity to acquire tolerance. The school nurse is often in a position to encounter firmly held views which are contrary to her own personal or professional beliefs and contrary to the objectives which she wishes to achieve. All the communication and persuasive skills are necessary to effect change(s) in this event.
3. Lack of bias, prejudice and being nonjudgemental are expected attitudes of health care practitioners. The first may be interpreted as lack of bias in matters which concern the privacy of individuals, but a commitment to create a bias towards positive health. Prejudice can present a difficulty or

dilemma. Where it is so ingrained that it is not amenable to change, it has to be overcome in professional life so that it does not affect others. Being nonjudgemental is one basis for providing effective health care. Professional judgement has to be based on facts and data and their interpretation and should relate to the issues which are the professional's responsibility. Other judgements should be avoided or deferred until all facts and opinions are known, and even then must be recognized as personal rather than factual or professional.

SUPPORT

Professionals often function in relative isolation and carry a burden of responsibility. They therefore require support, but must also be prepared to *provide* support. An effective support system is a tool of professional practice. The health care worker, in this instance the school nurse, should provide support for her clientele, their parents, their teachers and other carers who may be involved. Support can have many facets; it may be practical or emotional, be required for short or long periods, and change its context or intensity. Support, while an essential ingredient, also has dangers in that it can lead to dependency on the one hand or over-commitment on the other. Supportive systems therefore require balance and constant re-consideration and review.

Apart from the support provided for clients (children), school nurses are mutually involved in three support systems:

1. Collegiate, involving the members of the various teams, people from one's own discipline and colleagues from other branches of nursing.
2. Managerial, in that there should be a formalized support network. It is often stated that 'management' must support its staff; I would like to suggest that any support system must have elements of mutuality.
3. Background, in that few professionals function in isolation and need the support of their families, friends and social circle.

SPACE AND FACILITIES

The most common problem encountered in current school nursing practice is the unavailability or unsuitability of rooms. According to regulations implementing the 1944 and 1948 Education Acts, which have never been repealed, each school catering for more than a minimum number of pupils, i.e. 98 per cent of schools currently in existence, should have a room regularly available for use by medical and allied personnel. The regulations also suggest that this room should have facilities for carrying out health care functions, and some facility for storing records and equipment. In reality, many schools and their governing bodies or responsible education authorities, have not provided this facility.

Modern schools, that is, schools built since the mid-1950s, have rooms which were designed for this purpose, but despite this the problem persists. It has been problematic for schools to consider leaving a room under-used when there has been excess pressure on all space. Few schools now have the same pressures, as the number of pupils has diminished in most places, but habits are hard to overcome. Nurses who, because of excessive case/ workloads, have visited 'their' schools infrequently or irregularly have rarely negotiated appropriate space for their use. This picture is changing rapidly, in that nurses are very aware that physical facilities must enable them to carry out their role and functions effectively, and that their responsibility includes the accuracy of screening procedures. Ill-suited rooms do not lend themselves to hearing or vision testing, and all children have the right to expect some measure of privacy when attending for health care interview or medical examination. Many schools have now made a room permanently available, and some nurses have provided a schedule when they will accept self-referrals or be available to provide advice at each of their schools.

If no suitable space can be found in the school building, such rooms will have to be sought in health centres or surgeries. The temporary departure of large groups of pupils or whole classes is much more disruptive to the school than the release of small groups of children to be seen on site.

The most amenable solution is to have negotiated access to a room which allows realistic and appropriate facility, the use of the room to be mutually agreed according to pressures of timetabling, and the nurse's work programme. As well as availability there are a few basic requirements of any space or room which is used for health care, assessment or medical procedures:

1. It should have sufficient length to allow vision testing, unless the test equipment is adaptable to room size.
2. It should be relatively free from loud and disruptive noises so that hearing testing can be accomplished.

3. It should be adequately lighted and aired, as well as reasonably warm, to facilitate health surveys.
4. It should have the facility, preferably lockable, to store equipment.
5. It should be free from interruptions so that privacy is assured.
6. It should be vacant and accessible as arranged to allow health care with minimum disruption to the school.

Ideally, and few places have reached this ideal, the room should be available to the nurse at all times, so that she can use it for teaching sessions, or for instituting such innovations as health clubs, relaxation or stress-releasing sessions, slimming clubs, discussion groups or any other session that may be necessary. The facility may be shared with the first-aider, who may wish to take advantage of the lock-up facilities, but it should not be confused with a first-aid room.

The room used by the nurse should be close to washing facilities, and preferably a wash basin should be within the room. It is likely that there will have to be frequent washing of hands when dealing with the personal care of children, and it may be necessary to use this facility, or persuade a child to use this facility, before being able to provide personal care.

EQUIPMENT

The equipment used by school nurses is not costly. In fact it is very cheap in comparison with the equipment used for curative measures. This may be one reason why it continues to be under-valued. In many instances there appear to be shortages of the most basic equipment, usually because little thought has been given to its provision, and very often because nurses have not requested it. Sometimes requests have been made and not met. This is usually because the request has been made verbally and not supported by written statements or because the reason for the request has not been stated clearly. Sometimes it is difficult to gain any budgetary allocation mid-year, and requests can take up to 18 months to reach fruition. Often the request has been ignored, because it has been so small that it did not appear to merit attention.

Assessment tools should match the nature of the assessments to be made. Many nurses continue to use hearing test equipment which is simple to use, and will only assess on a superficial level. A range of machinery has been developed to lead to accurate determination of details of pitch and range and thereby to assessment of need. Most of this machinery is not complex, and its use can be learned in a very short time with very little practice. Greater skill is required in interpreting the readings of the machine, but again this is an easily acquired skill. In many places nurses work in partnership with audiometricians, the nurse doing the preliminary, rough scan of a whole school population, the audiometrician testing the children who are suspected of some degree of hearing loss. Hearing loss can be minimal or profound, temporary and amenable to treatment, or permanent. There may be a loss in one register of sound only, or through a range of sounds. The nurse's role in profound loss is to act as a referral agent; in minimal or temporary hearing loss she is the person who initiates treatment and ensures that reassessment occurs. It may be essential to discover the underlying causes, which could be repeated colds, catarrh, malnutrition, or over-exposure to continuous loud noise. The nurse may also be instrumental in ensuring that the child does not suffer educationally through hearing loss by informing the teacher and suggesting that the child should be better placed in the classroom to hear instructions (ACSHIP, 1979; Thomas, 1985).

Vision testing

Vision testing is another 'bread and butter' part of the nurse's work. There are only two kinds of professionals who are inherently more skilled at this task, i.e. consultant ophthalmologists and opticians. The first are not always available and waiting lists may be long, with specific attentions to those who require intensive or lengthy treatments, or have diseases such as diabetes, which may lead to loss of vision. The second are usually locally based, with easy access, but some people, especially children, are reluctant to make realistic use of this facility. It is therefore the nurse's function to persuade all those who would benefit to use the opticians' services and skills, and equally it is important to ensure, in co-operation with teachers and parents, that prescribed glasses are worn, broken glasses mended and that children do not feel disadvantaged or get teased by having to wear spectacles. This function sounds so simple until one attempts to fulfil it! Broken, pocketted instead of worn, distorted and ill-fitting glasses represent a permanent nightmare, especially among young, sports-loving boys.

The school nurse usually scan tests the whole school population, at intervals commensurate with the policy of her employing authority. The first criterion for enabling a successful scan is to ensure that the test equipment, however simple, is suitable for use in the space provided. Each of the letter or picture charts normally used specifies the distance at which it is most effective. Many scans have proved invalid, or have floundered because the distance between child and chart tester were wrong, and either have had to be repeated or led to missing children in need of attention. If the space used is the same at all times, markers can be placed to avoid repetition of this problem. If the available space changes, new distance measurements will have to be taken at the start of each session.

Some vision scans have proved to be invalid because the light in the space used was such that children were prevented from seeing the charts without distortion. The nurse must ensure that lighting is adequate for the purpose. Daylight is most desirable, but good artificial light can be equally effective.

In some instances it is essential to discuss with teachers the state of the child's or children's knowledge of letters, so that vision testing can be adapted from letters to pictures, or from specific letters to letter shapes.

It is helpful, especially with small children, to have assistance while testing, to that they can be helped to cover one eye, or to be reassured when they apparently do not perform to expectations. Knowledge of child development is also essential: children's vision undergoes changes with increasing age, and some children may reach their peak at a different rate than others. It was thought at one time that children reached perfect visual acuity very early in infancy; this has proved erroneous (Bee, 1981). Assistance with testing is also beneficial, though not essential, with older children. They do love to partially remove any eye-covering, play around and not attend to the matter in hand. Parents, teachers, colleagues, prefects and students or trainees could all fall into the helper category.

Testing for colour discernment has to be undertaken at the appropriate time. It is crucial for some older pupils, who have career aspirations which require perfect colour vision, becoming a pilot for example, to become aware of any deficiency as early as possible, and certainly to enable counselling and support. The support is vital, as some youngsters are extremely disappointed and distressed to find that they are less than perfect, even though it is a matter outwith anyone's control. Counselling may occur at several levels, but perhaps the most urgent may be careers advice and an appropriate choice of examination subjects. Parents may be anxious to know the outcome of such a test if there is any history of colour-blindness in the family. For some children it may explain a difficulty in such subjects as art, or their rather different dress sense from that of their peers. Like vision itself, colour vision develops through childhood, starting with a differentiation of broad bands of colours, leading to finer recognition and lastly the naming of colours. Some children are able to differentiate clearly, but never learn to name. There is some difference of opinion among experts regarding the stage of development when colour vision is complete. It would seem, on balance, that children of eight or nine years can differentiate broadly, whereas few children below the age of 12 can differentiate completely. By the age of 13 all children should be able to recognize all colours, even if they do not know their names (Brown, 1978).

The most commonly used test continues to be the Ishihara (Illingsworth, 1975), which is in book form and easily transportable, as well as being adaptable for close or distance use. This spans broad and fine elements, and can be used to assess a whole class or school, or used on occasion with any individual either to ascertain development or to reassure. There is nothing to prevent the book being used as often as the nurse deems it necessary, the one proviso being that such a tool forms part of her readily available equipment.

Both vision and hearing of the testers, i.e. the school nurses, should be checked regularly, at least every two years, and steps taken to overcome any deficits, as recommended by the DHSS in their response to the ACSHIP report in 1981 (DHSS, 1981, Social Services Sub-Committee, para 3–2–5). Such testing can be carried out as a collegiate exercise or as part of management policy; in either event it is essential to enable competent practice.

Weight and height

Measuring weight and height are essentials for ascertaining physical development and/or the absence of disease. Many young children will cease to grow when they suffer from emotional distress, so the physical measurements can be indicators of a range of difficulties. Such measurements, however, are less than useful when they occur in isolation. They should be charted or otherwise recorded at regular intervals and compared with expected norms.

However, it seems too obvious to reiterate that scales are needed for measuring weight. It is a sad fact that many scales in current use do not provide accurate measurements. They are either damaged, ill maintained, or buried by so much clutter that they are impossible to adjust. Whether the instrument in use is a modern, sensitive one or an older variety, whether it registers digitally or in notches, whether it provides information in grammes and kilogrammes or stones and ounces, accuracy should be assured. This requires protective storage, away from the onslaught of games or intentional damage, an even floor surface for the time it is in use, and regular balancing by the firm who originally supplied it or by the employer's maintenance division. The type of scale which has to be transported from place to place, even room to room, is more prone to maladjustment than one placed securely in a guaranteed base.

In the same vein, it seems too obvious to need stating that a reliable gauge is needed for measuring height. Many types of devices can be seen: these include pictorial guides provided by some firms who wish to draw attention to their product; notches on walls; measures attached to scales, tape-measures attached to walls; and hand-held devices. The accuracy of many of the measurements taken with volatile tools is of doubtful merit. It is essential to use a calibrated, firmly positioned tool of adequate length, as well as ensuring that the person to be measured is standing properly, on a level surface and without distortion by heeled shoes.

Low stature may be of concern. If persistent or regressive, it may indicate malnutrition, hormonal malfunction, several diseases caused by malnutrition or hormone deficiency, or signs of neglect or abuse. If measurements are not accurate or if they are undervalued and badly recorded, referral for treatment may be delayed and early signs missed, so that a disease becomes a handicap instead of responding to treatment.

There are some people who will be of low stature due to hereditary factors, such as children born to parents from parts of Japan. However, it is dangerous to assume that all Japanese children will be of short stature. The same applies to any ethnic grouping where short stature predominates. All measurements should be relative to each other, applied to individual children, and show a rate of progression. It is the halt in progress, or a drop in stature, however minimal, which is the indicator lending itself to preventive and protective action.

Growth spurts are part of normal development, and therefore any recording of height will not follow a perfectly straight line. Some children do exceed height expectations. A few of these will require specialist attention, as again this may portend serious hormonal problems. Many will require support and reassurance, as excessive tallness can be as distressing as excessive smallness. Teasing, the formation of boy–girl relationships and fear of further continuous growth often form the mainstream of concerns.

Measuring devices are being improved and developed, and the best source of information is the Child Growth Foundation (2 Mayfair Avenue, London W1 1PW; tel. 01–995 0267). Charts provided by companies can form the background in support of the nurse's activities. They can be placed so that children can follow their own progress and development, so that they create an interest in healthy eating for development and generally can be used as teaching tools.

Teaching and demonstration materials form another large group of essential equipment needed by school nurses. Being an expert on health matters does not mean that one can explain these without the assistance of a range of materials. Some of these may be readily available in any school, such as textbooks, project materials and a human atlas. However, the nurse may need to search for the most appropriate materials; some indication of where to find these is given in the reference following Chapter 11. The easiest and handiest of teaching materials are inherent in the assessment tools used and discussed above.

Children learn more eagerly when they can relate this to themselves and, when explained and illustrated by charts, the records of their own development can form a useful base-line. Demonstration materials are somewhat different. Bandages and similar equipment used when teaching the principles of first-aid are one sort of demonstration equipment; live infants used when teaching parentcraft may be regarded differently. The first can be adapted to any situation, the second requires close ethical and practical considerations. Whichever materials are used, the nurse must be very familiar with them, and have practised handling them in public. It is easy to dress an infant after its bath when you are a nurse, parent or grandparent; it is quite difficult to do the same when there are 20 pairs of curious eyes watching you and when you have to watch the possessors of those eyes, as well as the infant you are handling, in case there is any distraction or mischief.

The nurse may require a range of other equipment, but this will vary according to the details of the job she is expected to perform, the policies for certain screening procedures within the district, the availability of equipment for loan to parents and to some extent her own expertise, specialized interests or the context and time at which her functions are performed. Such tools may include: enuresis pads and bells; sphygmomanometers; urinalysis kits; specialized measuring devices; exercise programmes; and diet information and charts.

One type of tool has received much debate, and that is the provision of protective clothing for the nurse herself. Few school nurses continue to wear uniforms or identifiable clothing. Despite this it is sometimes interesting to see how many can be identified anywhere by, for example, the standard issue bag, usually bulging at its seams. Most of the time it would be counterproductive to wear any uniform. In some settings, and in many situations, it is desirable to wear a protective covering such as an overall. Many employing authorities provide these and make provision or allowance for their laundry. In some instances nurses have to request issue or permission to purchase such clothes, and negotiate responsibility for replacement, laundry or allowance to accomplish either or both.

First-aid equipment may be required by those nurses who combine their school health functions with that of first-aider, or those who are responsible for training the first-aid assistants for any school setting. It seems important that the nurse, whichever of the above may be her remit, is aware of the advances in materials used, such as for example burns dressings, and that she ensures the equipment is adequate and reasonably maintained. She may need to advise on the setting up of such equipment, and on its variability in those settings where there is a concentration on sports, as compared to those where there is a concentration on laboratories and workshops. As well as working with the first-aider, she may have to negotiate with health and safety representatives from both the education authority and the trades unions.

RECORDS AND THEIR SAFE STORAGE

Records and their importance have been mentioned several times, and related to many aspects of the school nurse's function and tools, and this theme will no doubt recur. *Records are essential tools for competent professional practice.* In recent years much work has been undertaken to make records into useful, finely honed tools, and in many places nurses have contributed to this work (DHSS and Welsh Development Agency, 1984–86). Much of confidentiality is a myth, though this does not obviate the necessity to create safe storage facilities. To be useful, records must be available to compare measurements, to assess the success or otherwise of care plans, to provide data on which to base resource allocation, including staff time, and to demonstrate effective, competent practice. The storage of these documents therefore becomes a matter which transcends the arguments of who should have access, but makes it important that they are kept both safe (undamaged) and accessible to all those who may have legitimate use for them. As an essential tool for the school nurse, they should be located in the school or so close to it that retrieval is not time-consuming; they should be safe, that is stored in a way which protects them as far as possible from floods, fire and vandalism; they should be of a nature which allows easy recording of all the relevant information, including percentile charts and pictorial or diagrammatic representation of other measurements; they should be legibly written or typewritten which may imply that there should be secretarial or computer resources to maintain them; and they should be completed immediately after use.

It should be decided at what stage they become accessible to the children whose health they record, or whether it may be preferable to maintain duplicate records, one held by the nurse or her employers and one by the child and its parents. Greater success has been reported when children have been made totally responsible for retaining their records and producing these on request and at need. They are then available for use by several professionals rather than being stored – and often mislaid – in official premises. Additionally, records should be transferable to other schools in other districts, and thus useful to health care workers wherever they may need to make use of them.

SUMMARY

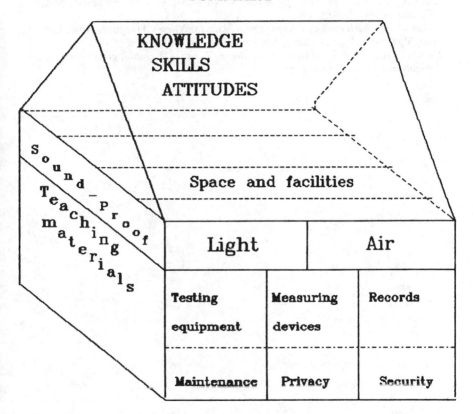

REFERENCES

Argyle, M. (1982) *The Psychology of Interpersonal Behaviour*, Penguin, London.
Ashworth, P. (1980) *Care to Communicate*, Royal College of Nursing, London.
ACSHIP (1979) *Report to DHSS by the Advisory Committee on Services for Hearing Impaired Children*, DHSS, London.
Bee, H. (1981) *The Developing Child*, Harper & Row, New York.
Brown, G. (1978) *Child Development*, Open Books Publishing, London.
DHSS and Welsh Development Agency (1984–86) *School Health Records*, DHSS, Cardiff.

Illingsworth, R.S. (1975) *The Normal School Child*, Churchill Livingstone, Edinburgh.

Interpersonal Skills – Continuing Nurse Education Programme (1986) A Self-Instruction Module. Available from Barnet College, 26 Danbury Street, London N1 8JU, or Central Manchester College, Openshaw Centre, Manchester M11 2WH.

Kagan, C.M. (ed.) (1985) *Interpersonal Skills in Nursing – Research and Application*, Croom Helm, Beckenham.

— *et al.* (1986) *A Manual of Interpersonal Skills for Nurses*, Harper & Row, London.

Satir, V. (1978) *Peoplemaking*, Souvenir Press, London.

Thomas, A.J. (1985) *Acquired Hearing Loss – Psychological Implications*, Academic Press, London.

7
EDUCATION AND TRAINING – THEORY

An introduction to *some* of the
theoretical components of the current syllabus.

The current syllabus for the Course in School Nursing was formulated in 1978 by the then Council for the Education and Training of Health Visitors (CETHV) following a five-year period of negotiations with the Departments of Health of the four UK countries, circulation of a draft syllabus and consultation with the profession. The present document is the result of the work of the CETHV's committees and the recommendations of a working group which included nurse managers of school health and practising school nurses.

The length of the course, 12 weeks *minimum*, was agreed as a compromise solution: managers stated it would be impossible to release nurses for longer periods; nurses were unsure or unable to demonstrate what they really required; and the CETHV anticipated that it would be possible in due course to incorporate this 12-week course into the 51-week health visitor course as a complete module. It was thought that this would open doors to career progression as well as avoid any serious splintering of the professional and status differentials. The English National Board (ENB) accepted the syllabus and its conditions, though it was evident by 1983 when the ENB was established, that the module idea had not been taken up, and that only a few of the 20 approved training courses were exceeding minimum requirements.

During 1979 to 1983, some 1,500 nurses successfully completed the course, and they clearly indicated that they considered the course content appropriate, but the time allocated to its completion inadequate. The demand for more in-depth study of the theory surrounding school nursing practice, and for increased practical experience as part of the course, has increased and become vocal, but as yet there has been no opportunity to negotiate change. However, it has been agreed tacitly that this is one of the syllabi which will receive attention, as a matter of urgency, once it becomes clear which aspects of the proposals currently with the profession for consultation, e.g. the Cumberlege Report (May, 1986) and Project 2000 (May, 1986), are accepted both by the profession and by government.

The similarities between many parts of this book and the syllabus are purely deliberate. Other parts represent those elements which it may not be possible to include in the 12 weeks of the course. The following paragraphs concentrate on those parts of the theoretical component which have not been covered elsewhere, and Chapter 8 looks at planned and assessed practice elements.

COURSE PLANNING

Each course in school nursing is proposed to the Statutory Body (ENB) by the Training Institution which intends to provide it. The criteria for approval of a course are clearly contained in the guide to the syllabus, the Rules as agreed by the UK Health Ministers and the Regulations and circulars of the National Boards detail the requirements for each course submission. No course is approved in perpetuity but each has to be re-submitted at least once in five years.

Course planning should take place in the months preceding the submission, and should be based on evaluations of previous courses, discussion with seconding authorities, employers, and with past and present students and their practice assessors. The syllabus is deliberately worded in a broad fashion, and should enable considerable developments at local levels. It lays down *minimum* requirements, but does not in any way block progress beyond this minimum. As in all situations there are constraints, such as the number of students likely to be seconded to the course, the education authority's requirement for viable numbers, the resources available for teaching and learning, and the pressures on the course members *vis-à-vis* their case/workloads and personal commitments, which may mitigate against certain course patterns.

There is little constraint on the pattern of a course, provided it can be shown that the proposals are both practicable and suitable. Existing courses follow a variety of patterns, including a 12-week block system, several short blocks, blocks interspersed with guided study, and day-release over an extended period. Evaluations have not demonstrated any marked variations in outcomes whichever pattern has been followed, except in the case of day-release programmes. These have appeared desirable as giving the student adequate time to assimilate new knowledge and skills, but this has generally been negated by the fact that those on day-release were rarely regarded as students by their employers and peers, and carried a full case/workload while studying for their qualification.

The major aim of the planning cycle is to facilitate developments, with contributions from all those concerned, and vesting responsibility for the provision of courses and content within the educational setting.

AIMS AND GOALS OF A COURSE

Both aims and goals are stated clearly in the syllabus (National Boards for Nursing, Midwifery and Health Visiting for England, Wales, Scotland and Northern Ireland, 1985), and remain valid.

Aims
1. To prepare nurses to work in the school health service as members of teams responsible for the health of the school child and the adolescent.
2. To give students the opportunity of enhancing their skills and of extending their understanding and knowledge of nursing within an educational setting.
3. To increase insight into the role of the school nurse.

Goals
1. To acquire the practical and organizational skills appropriate to the work of the school nurse, including the ability to identify and assess needs for work within the school health service.
2. To relate knowledge of normal growth and development to the physical, psychological, social and intellectual needs of schoolchildren and adolescents.
3. To increase the ability to recognize significant deviations from the norm, in order to be able to initiate appropriate action.
4. To extend knowledge of the health and education services in the community, and the social context in which school nurses function.
5. To develop skills of communication and interpersonal relationships, in order to become an effective member of an interdisciplinary team.

It is evident that goals could be extended almost indefinitely, and that they could be expressed in behavioural terms, e.g. 'at the end of the course the student will be able to . . .', or in terms of models of learning which could help to make course outcomes successful, but which are likely to be open to misinterpretation, or at least variable interpretation. The present syllabus, its aims and goals, have remained valid because it is expressed in clear, unequivocal everyday English. Any extension can therefore concentrate on meeting the educational needs of nurses of the late 1980s and 1990s, and incorporate advances in knowledge and skills.

One statement made in the introduction to the syllabus remains very significant, namely that courses should be sited in proximity to other related courses. The implicit intent is that all students should experience shared learning with those who may constitute team members of the future (or present), e.g. teachers, health visitors and trainee doctors. In reality, course planning or resource constraints have led to some courses being provided in relative isolation. It would appear that this is a matter requiring most urgent amelioration, possibly in the context of course development.

Section 1 of the syllabus, entitled 'School Nursing', is the most important, as exemplified in its 17 subheadings and their subparagraphs. It is noteworthy that this is Section 1, as compared with some related syllabi, e.g. health visiting, where Section 5 of that syllabus is the major element.

The other sections are also important, but as supporting and enhancing ones. Each of the subheadings can be extended and adapted to incorporate changes of knowledge base, practice or philosophy.

One omission appears to be ethical considerations related to practice. Professional ethics form a back-cloth for each practitioner and each caring team. They include philosophies of care, health policies and politics, issues of personal freedom versus intervention, child protection versus child rights; the need for a research base for practice versus the need to safe-guard client privacy. Each working day appears to present some situation which could be related to ethics. The UKCC has based its *Code of Professional Practice*, and the subsequent booklets dealing with Advertising and the Administration of Medicines on ethical considerations (UKCC, 1984, 1985, 1986). In its booklet, *Administration of Medicines*, the giving of advice as part of professional practice is considered as being on a par with the physical administration of the substances themselves. Therefore it is extremely relevant to those working in the community, including nurses working in educational settings. Nursing ethics have become the subject of recent study and report (Campbell, 1980). Additionally, many health authorities have now established ethics committees to give consideration to any proposal, such as research, which could contravene ethical boundaries, and to ensure as far as possible that clients are not subjected knowingly to unjustifiable pressures.

PRIORITIES AND ORGANIZATION OF WORK

Each working day, and throughout professional life, one is faced with the dilemma of determining and rationalizing priorities. Decisions can only be reached in full knowledge of all the parameters surrounding the situation, including health authority policies and availability of related services. The most important element is that priorities are not static; they must be reviewed regularly and amended. There is one major danger in prioritizing, namely that equally important 'routine' matters may continue to be regarded as less important until they reach the stage of constituting an omission. It is also important to ensure that the professional's priorities match those of the client or client group. Often there is a mismatch, created by a communication gap. Decisions about priorities should be clearly stated, and the relationship of these to other elements of the work defined.

Priorities can change for many reasons, including achievement of original objectives or care plans, alterations in the patterns of health and disease, sudden crises, demographic variations and new knowledge or enhanced practice. Work organization, while essential on a daily as well as a long-term basis, must be sufficiently flexible to accommodate changes. Such organization is first and foremost the responsibility of individual practitioners, who should be able to demonstrate competence in this arena.

Second, it may involve colleagues whose work impinges and, third, it is likely to relate to service managers who will seek assurance that workloads and caseloads are adequately covered.

Subsumed under organization of work are vital facets of management of change and of time. Management of change is a skill needed in most professional practice, and includes strategies for coping with differences and difficulties, mechanisms for personal and collective actions, the means of acquiring new and revised information which may lead to change and predicting the effects. Such predictions should be based on available evidence and attempt to incorporate as many factors and variables as possible.

Time management is a subject which is attracting much attention; it relates to cost-effectiveness, competence and accountability. Improved time management can reduce stress to positive levels, i.e. provide stimulation rather than stagnation, and can strengthen arguments for appropriate resources. The concept of time management gained currency with the increased pressures of shorter working hours, extensive needs and demands, and accelerated rates of change. It now forms a module of many management courses and is the subject of some intensive study by researchers. To date, research has resulted in a greater awareness of the need for efficient management of time, but does not appear to have provided many helpful answers.

INTERVIEWING AND COUNSELLING SKILLS

The conduct of sessions in schools, be they health surveys, health care interviews, medical examinations or health teaching, implies the acquisition and effective use of interviewing skills. Communication skills can provide the umbrella under which this is considered.

Interviewing skills are the art of structuring encounters to elicit relevant information in a non-threatening way with minimal intrusion into privacy, and yet providing the opportunity to incorporate discussion of all relevant issues. They presuppose that the interviewer knows and has indicated the parameters of the session, that objectives have been clarified before the start of any interview, and that there are implicit or explicit limits to the encounter. They also imply that the purpose of the interview is clear to all the parties involved, and that any subsequent action is a matter for decision and mutual agreement. They require appropriate use of language and recording systems, but do not ignore the underlying inhibitions and constraints affecting participants in any interview situation. Part of the skill is to clarify the components of the interaction which are likely to remain confidential to the participants, those which may be included in a broad analysis of a situation without divulging personal details, and those which are likely to be identifiable with the provider of the information. They must be based on mutual respect and trust. No successful interview can ignore nonverbal clues.

Often the quality of the interaction depends on the relative proximity of participants, their physical distance from each other, and the facility for eye-contact or other encouragements. Gestures, which are not reflected in any written record, can form one of the bases of a successful interview. Included in gestures are smiles, touch or other tactile stimuli, and consciousness, perhaps control, of involuntary reactions such as raised eyebrows, grimaces or disapproving tone of voice. In some interview situations language may need to be assisted by other forms of explanation to ensure that there is mutual understanding; diagrams, models, pictures and repetition in different ways are all part of the battery of skills.

The interviewer must be aware of the skills brought to the session by the interviewee, such as providing the answers that he imagines are required or would sound pleasing, the means to respond in a way which can distort or confuse the word-picture, and occasionally deliberate attempts to mislead.

The interviewee may provide nonverbal clues at variance with the spoken words and create an ambiance of either friendliness and acceptance, or distancing. Time management should be applied to any interview situation.

During a course of training, interviewing skills should be practised within the theoretical framework and during planned practice. Many institutions can provide facilities which allow self-assessment of performance on tape or screen, or which may include peer discussion. It needs constant practice, self-assessment and review to perfect techniques. One essential ingredient for successful interviewing appears to be presentation of self in a positive, honest and natural way.

Counselling skills are more intensive and targetted than generalized interviewing. No course in school nursing aims to prepare people as qualified counsellors, but courses usually aim to define the limits which exist between reacting appropriately to a situation or request, which may include some basic counselling, and in-depth, long-term and complex interaction which forms the basis of counselling as a strategy, treatment or therapy. School nurses should be aware of the extent and limitations of their skills, either on completion of training or following experience, and the point when they should act as a referral agent for counselling. The most important skill is to recognize the need for intensive counselling when it presents, to be able to assess the type of input required (practical, spiritual, subject-specific, emotional or psychological) and refer appropriately with minimal time-lapse. Some nurses may be involved in counselling as members of a team, in that they play a supporting role in the intervals between more intensive sessions; often they may need to follow-up the outcomes of referred actions and reassess whether additional or alternative actions are required.

All nurses should be health counsellors, able to discuss matters relating to the maintenance and promotion of health at the depth and detail relevant to a given situation. The implications are that their knowledge of health matters is extensive, up-to-date and applicable.

Both interviewing and counselling skills presume that listening skills have been acquired successfully, and are being enhanced with use. Interpretative skills often form part of the total pattern.

CARE AND STORAGE OF DRUGS AND MEDICINES

With the advent of integration of all pupils into normal schools, the range of medicines likely to be found in any school will become more diverse and extensive. Parents, and children once they are old enough, are responsible for the administration of prescribed medicines of all kinds. However, during the school day the head-teacher stands *in loco parentis*, i.e. a parent substitute. It can therefore be argued that any medication which has to be administered during the course of normal school hours becomes the responsibility of the teaching staff. Most medicines which have to be taken during this time are likely to be of a temporary nature, and there is likely to be a time limit on their efficacy. Some children will require continued treatments at regular intervals. Those in the educational setting face several problems as a result, and the school nurse may have to be instrumental in providing the advice which leads to safe practice.

The first issue is the actual administration of medicines, or if it involves an older child, supervision so that essential drug maintenance is not forgotten with the possibility of disastrous consequences. Generally speaking, teachers do not consider themselves competent to handle medicines or drugs, and whenever possible make arrangements with parents towards mutually satisfactory solutions. There are instances when this is not possible, and teachers may be required to deal with the situation. In most instances, especially if this consists of a reminder that, for example, it is time for tablets to be taken, the teacher will see that the right number of such tablets are swallowed, and/or that suitable liquid is available to facilitate this. If teachers should be required to actually hand out the substances, instructions regarding this may have to be given in each case. Additionally, each teacher will wish to clarify their responsibility, which does not usually include knowledge of dosages or drugs. The most expedient solution is for each child to bring a measured daily supply, separated and labelled into component parts, so that the teacher's responsibility ends with ascertaining that the correct portion has been imbibed. The complexity increases when medicines are other than tablets. It is unlikely that teachers' roles will incorporate the giving of injections or the measuring of liquid dosages, and arrangements will have to be made for this to be achieved by other means. In the 'normal' range of schools, nurses are not able to take on this role, as they will be on more than one site, and not regularly available. The person on site who is trained in first-aid is generally likely to be less competent to act than the classroom teacher.

The second problem is the safe storage of prescribed medicines and drugs. Two facets are particularly important: storage at required temperatures, especially for those medicines which must be kept hot or cold; and protection from abuse by other children. Many pills can be mistaken for sweets, or experimentation can appear attractive to youngsters. Schools will therefore have to devise a means of overcoming the storage problem. The medical or first-aid rooms seem to be ideally suited to provide such facility, but arrangements for access by those responsible for the daily supervision and administration will have to be made and clearly communicated. The nurse should play an active advisory role in this.

The third problem is knowledge of the effects and side-effects of medicines. Few teachers will wish to know the detailed composition of drugs, nor their healing properties, but they may insist on knowing what would happen if dosage is omitted at any time, or what changes in behaviour, attention span or ability they can expect, immediately following the taking of medicines or during the child's time at school. Each school nurse can legitimately be expected to provide some of the answers to teachers' questions, and equally importantly know where to obtain such information speedily. This implies a regular revision of knowledge acquired during nurse education and training, and regular updating to keep abreast of developments. Few people, even professionals, can be *au fait* with all current medicines and treatments; there are frequent and profound changes. Nurses should, however, have access to such information through their health authority or medical colleagues.

Some children will nowadays be integrated into normal schools though they require a range of on-site treatments, examples may be stoma care or suction. It is unrealistic to expect a teacher who has responsibility for many children to cope with such specialisms, nor the school nurse or health visitor who are in the school for specified periods only. Arrangements for dealing with these matters have to be made on individual bases; these can include employment of care attendants – possibly instructed and supervised by the school nurse – or regular and repeated access by informal carers, usually relatives of the child. One of the school nurse's increasing roles may be to assist the child in gaining as much independence as possible.

Nurses who work in special schools are likely to deal with drugs and treatments on a regular basis; how this is achieved will depend on the nature and size of the school, and the overall workload of the nurse.

HUMAN DEVELOPMENT

School nursing practice should be based on a sound theoretical framework The basis for undertaking developmental screening and assessment is a knowledge of human development, specifically as applied to children of school age. It is important that the factors which lead to optimum health on school entry and school leaving are recognized, and also those which form the basis for healthy adulthood. There are many detailed texts which seek to describe child development; their range shows the complexity of the subject. Those by Erikson (1973) and Hadfield (1970) are just two examples of the many published.

One factor affecting development is nutrition. Many texts have been written setting out to describe the essentials of nutrition and nutritional values; it sometimes seems as though new ones reach the shelves daily, some contradicting previously established information. Nurses need to be aware of the current state of knowledge, issues being debated, and develop the ability to assess reports for their intrinsic and practical value (Koch, 1981; DHSS, 1983). In addition to the school nurse's role of knowing about personal care, she must also know about nutrition and be able to use such knowledge to form the basis of health teaching, or to establish care plans for those with diet-related needs. Nutritional content needs to differentiate between proven facts and information, and vogues or fads, as well as unsubstantiated ideas. Media influences on ideas about nutrition are fairly pervasive, and have to be treated similarly to those contained in some reports. The influence of glossy magazines and television are extensive.

There are other factors which can affect development and the potential for learning and achieving at school. Knowledge and understanding of the influence of environment, of psychological and emotional development, and factors which may inhibit or enhance this should all be part of school nurse education, at qualifying and post-qualification levels.

INTRODUCTION TO SOCIOLOGY AND SOCIAL PSYCHOLOGY

This section of the syllabus attempts to distil relevant material for school nursing practice from an extensive and increasing body of knowledge. In the context of a short (12-week) course, little more than a whetting of the appetite for discovering more about these subjects can be achieved. Seven areas of relevance are listed in the official syllabus (National Boards, 1985); it could equally be 17.

It has become increasingly important for all health care professionals to gain an understanding of the social structure in which they function, as well as an appreciation that this situation is far from static. The composition of families, roles within the family, the significance of being an eldest or youngest child, or a member of a large sibling group, and the possible significance of extended families and kinship groups may each affect the way in which health care for children and young people can be effective. It will certainly affect the deliverance and acceptability of services. Most modern societies, and certainly society within the cities of the UK, are composed of members of disparate cultural and religious groups. The values and ethics of each group will be significant to the ways in which they behave and the nature of health care which they demand and find acceptable, including dietary advice. Each group will have fundamental ideas related to health, and care plans should be formulated in the knowledge that they do not transgress cultural mores.

It is also important that nurses recognize that an educational setting is in fact a social organism, and that each setting functions as a total system, responding to external and internal stimuli. The social system of each school slots into other systems in its environment and will relate to these either harmoniously or be in conflict with them. An element of conflict can lead to positive developments, acrimonious conflict can create additional stress. The school nurse may be involved in encouraging developments, or assisting in defusing conflict. Many volumes, from paperbacks to tomes, have been written, only three are mentioned in the references as providing an overview of relevance in this context (Cotgrove, 1967; Gaffin, 1981; Walwin, 1982). The difficulty in selecting references, or further reading of interest, occurs because new researches are published frequently, and each professional practitioner has to make decisions as to their application and relevance. The newest branch of sociology, though even this is now more than a decade old, is the sociology of health and illness. Its most pertinent contributions to the body of knowledge are concepts relating to the roles taken by patients/ clients and the interfaces between different social systems (Tuckett, 1976).

SOCIAL POLICY

The qualifying course for school nurses can only provide an introduction to the ways in which social policies are formed and how they can be affected by practice and practitioners. It will also provide insight into the parameters in which school nurses function, such as the NHS, the education service, other caring agencies, financial provision and benefit entitlements. None of these are static entities, and there has to be continual updating of information throughout professional life. The course should also provide an outline of the legal framework which applies to nursing in educational settings, and explore the roles and functions of other members of the various teams to whom school nurses relate.

It is desirable that philosophies relating to health care and educational need are explored, but there may be insufficient time in current courses to do justice to this interesting and wide field.

This section of the syllabus has the most profound relevance for the future, as it should clarify that social policies can be affected and changed, and that each person may have a role in creating a climate for change, as well as being active as an instrument of change. It could lead to continuing and stimulating debate regarding the nurse's role as an agent of change, and the influence which can be exerted at individual or group levels. Concern is often expressed that interest in and knowledge of these issues, philosophies and parameters could lead to political actions. All policies are based on politics, whether at local or national levels, and nurses urgently need to become politically aware. This does not refer to membership of any political party; it should be each person's free choice whether they wish to be affiliated in any way; but to knowing when, where and how to influence any system, the implications of such influence and the implications if no influence is brought to bear. It also means knowing how, when and by whom decisions are made, and to take an active part in decision-making processes (Salvage, 1985; White, 1985).

ATTITUDE CHANGE

Each course participant will bring sets of values, beliefs and attitudes gained through their particular life and work experiences. Some of these may be profoundly challenged, others may be reinforced. It is clear that due to the short period of the course, challenges can prove both stimulating and painful, that desirable change may become apparent but that any process of attitude or belief change is likely to be incomplete at the end of a 12-week period. It is therefore helpful, or even essential, that newly qualified practitioners have the opportunity to continue the change or learning process. The course may equip them to re-examine the foundations of their individual practice, such as attitudes, at regular intervals; the facility to do so should be created throughout professional life.

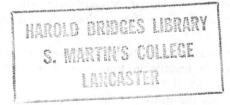

SUMMARY

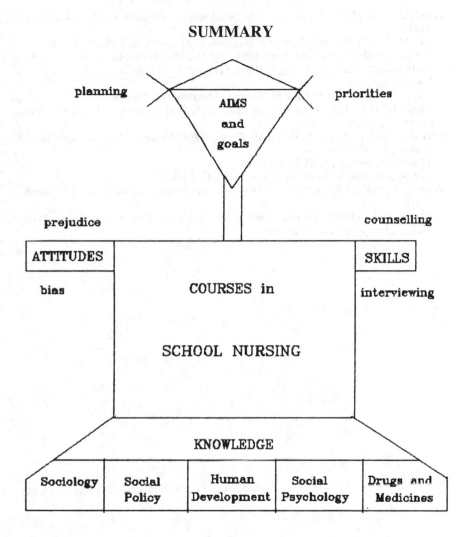

REFERENCES

Campbell, A.V. (1980) *Moral Dilemmas in Medicine*, Churchill Livingstone, Edinburgh.
Cotgrove, S. (1967) *The Science of Society – An Introduction to Sociology*, Allen & Unwin, London.
DHSS (1983) *Manual of Nutrition*, HMSO, London.
Erikson, E. (1973) *Childhood and Society*, Penguin Books, Harmondsworth.
Gaffin, J. (1981) *The Nurse and The Welfare State*, H.M. & M., Aylesbury, Bucks.

Hadfield, J.A. (1970) *Childhood and Adolescence,* Penguin Books, Harmondsworth.

Koch, M. (1981) *The Whole Health Handbook,* Sidgwick & Jackson, London.

National Boards for Nursing, Midwifery and Health Visiting for England, Wales, Scotland and Northern Ireland (1985) *Syllabus for a Course in School Nursing,* UKCC, London.

Salvage, J. (1985) *The Politics of Nursing,* Heinemann, London.

Tuckett, D. (ed.) (1976) *An Introduction to Medical Sociology,* Tavistock Publications, London.

UKCC (1984) *Code of Professional Practice for Nurses, Midwives and Health Visitors,* UKCC, London.

— (1985) *Advertising,* UKCC, London.

— (1986) *Administration of Medicines,* UKCC, London.

Walwin, J. (1982) *A Social History of English Childhood,* Pelican Books, Harmondsworth.

White, R. (ed.) (1985) *Political Issues in Nursing: Past, Present and Future,* Wiley Medical Publications, Chichester.

8
EDUCATION AND TRAINING – PRACTICE

An interpretation of practice elements
of the current syllabus.

The current syllabus for a Course in School Nursing approved by the National Boards for Nursing, Midwifery and Health Visiting (1985) of all four United Kingdom countries states that practical experience, which is planned, assessed and supervised, is an integral part of the course. The guidance to syllabus interpretation acknowledges that those entering the courses may have extensive or minimal experience in the school health field and that this experience is likely to have varied in quantity and quality. The assessment of such experience is complex, the assessed student being dependent on the guidance she obtains from the supervisor and assessor. A dilemma is encountered by those who have been in employment as school nurses for any length of time and are assessed as needing additional practice before completing the course and being eligible to record their qualification with the UKCC. The longer the period of service prior to the assessment, the greater the dilemma. The syllabus indicates, rather than specifies, the areas in which each nurse should have assessed experience, but gives freedom to the training institution to select those areas which may need most attention for any individual. The selection of students is therefore a crucial factor, at which decisions can be made about existing competencies, and those which need to be acquired during the course.

Some of the practice elements which form the basis of school nursing are considered in other chapters and contexts. The procedures followed by nurses in some of their practice are considered in detail in the book by Nash (1985) and are not repeated here. The following paragraphs concentrate on those aspects which are still a matter for some debate and which should be given very close attention when the time comes to develop, extend or amend the present syllabus.

HEALTH SURVEYS

Current practice is variable, but in essence schoolchildren receive at least three major health checks during their school career, namely on school entry, school change and school leaving. There has been a move from thorough physical and psychological examination of each pupil towards survey by selective sampling and questionnaire, or reliance on previous information and referral. This move places increasing onus on the knowledge and skills of the school nurse in carrying out the selection of pupils for full examination and in making decisions which could affect the health of the population for which she carries responsibility. The debate about which is the best service, either selective mechanisms and sampling or examination of each person, has never been resolved, and substantive evidence is scarce. It does seem that it is essential to base any determination of health care needs on more evidence than can be acquired by questionnaire, but whether this necessitates examination of each pupil remains questionable.

Children can be referred for an examination or health check at any time during school life, the referral agent being any adult in contact with or otherwise concerned about the child. In those instances where nurses have become known to and accepted by their clientele, and especially where they are regularly accessible, self-referral by pupils old enough to do so becomes part of the pattern. Ideally, self-referral should be encouraged and backed by facilities to act upon such referral without undue time-lapse. Effective self-referral is usually based on increasing knowledge of bodily function acquired during health education input, as well as the interpersonal relationship formed between pupil and professional. In each instance the nurse has to use her professional judgement about the need for further action, the level of support, advice or counselling she can provide, and the need for specialist or other professional input. Many of the self-referral situations require difficult decisions, which can only be made on individual bases, including whether the matter can be kept confidential, whether it can be discussed with other members of the education or health care teams, or whether it is essential to alert parents or guardians.

Any health survey should be a team effort. The base-line is information received from previous records, teachers, parents and the child. Diagnostic skills and expertise should be provided by the school medical officer or a specialist such as an educational psychologist. The school nurse contributes special expertise based on assessment procedures. The DHSS has issued some guidelines about assessments and health surveys during school life, but these are a recommendation and not a directive (DHSS, 1978).

Health surveys should indicate health education needs, and can provide the opportunity for personalized health teaching. One very important feature of any health survey is the information this provides about the health status of the school, the community and how this compares with other communities, towns or countries. It should indicate macro health care needs, as opposed to the individual needs of children and families.

The nurse has an important role in analysing available data. The current era of basing resource allocation and formulating policies on the basis of such data makes this a crucial element of her practice. An analysis of assessments and measurements for each age-group, school or schools contained within a district should demonstrate trends in health, patterns of debility and need, and dramatic changes or rates of change. It should lead to realistic estimates of the kind of service which may be required in the future. This type of analysis is complementary to, and may form part of, analyses of immunization and vaccination uptakes, patterns of disease and handicap and of existing service provision. The last type of analysis is usually undertaken centrally, while the first has to be initiated at local levels and co-ordinated on a broader basis.

Analyses should demonstrate past achievements, which are most easily seen in reductions in infectious diseases, accidents and addictions. They should also incorporate the achievements of individual practitioners or groups of staff: such as evaluations of teaching sessions; the incidence of minor or temporary hearing loss which has been prevented from developing into disability or handicap; referral rates and the outcomes of referrals; success of care plans preventing obesity and other conditions; and any activities which merit attention.

HEALTH CARE INTERVIEWS

Health surveys and checks provide only a spasmodic and often selective coverage of the school-aged population. It is obvious that needs and crises arise in intervening periods, and that such irregular contact mitigates against getting to know children as individual people or establishing effective interpersonal relationships with them. By effective relationships is meant the building of trust and mutual respect which could create a climate, leading to health-enhancing behaviour changes, and acceptance of health teaching, advice and counselling. The named nurse being regularly on site and available is one means of creating this climate. Another means, found to be most effective where it has become established, is to offer regular health care interviews. Various time-scales have been debated and tried, the one found most practicable and effective is an annual interview with each child, apart from any referral and self-referral. Such an interview would include consideration of the physical, psychological, emotional and social needs of each child, and give both child and nurse the facility and opportunity to raise questions, concerns and points for discussion. The basis for each interview could vary from established routine, prior assessment and discerned health need, to referral to the nurse by a teacher, parent, doctor, health visitor, voluntary worker or professional from another agency.

Initially, health care interviews are likely to be lengthy as they will lay the foundations for future actions. Subsequent interviews will vary in length, depth and content. Interviews on a regular basis enable health care plans to be developed, agreed and acted upon.

A health care plan should set objectives to be achieved by the child, either independently or with the help of parents, teachers and nurse. It should state the means by which the objectives are to be achieved and build in reviews and rewards. The last may be self-satisfaction by the child, even a kind of bragging, at achieving the set goals. The nurse's contribution may be to monitor achievement and to provide the verbal rewards at seeing progress.

ATTENDANCE AT MEDICAL EXAMINATIONS

Many school nurses attend medical examinations but their role in this situation is not always clear, nor has it sometimes been sufficiently discussed, questioned or agreed. It is quite evident that the nurse's role should be a positive one. Usually she will know the child or children, she will have assessed their development and measured, recorded and analysed the criteria required for assessment purposes; in many instances she will have referred the child for thorough medical examination. In the latter case she should explain the reasons for requiring the assessment, and expect to be informed of the outcomes and proposed action. As an equal member of the health care team, she should be involved in the discussion about appropriate action or in the revision of health care plans following the assessment. The active contribution made by the nurse is likely to depend on the qualifications, expertise and experience of the medical officer with whom she is working. Some school medical officers are well-qualified in paediatrics and educational medicine and have great interest and experience in all matters relating to child health; others may be qualified but relatively inexperienced. Recently, some general medical practitioners have acquired a child health remit relating to school health. Among this group are those who are as qualified and able as the first-mentioned school medical officers, but there are others who have been steeped for many years in curative medicine and who find adapting to public and school health extremely difficult. Some of the latter are not familiar with procedures, some have only minimal experience of educational medicine and few have clear knowledge of the roles and functions of other members of educational and health teams.

The nurse's role is that of a professional person, a team member, who has clear lines of accountability and responsibility, who is expert in health, not medical, knowledge and who is equal but not subservient to another member of the team. She may have to act, as many ward sisters do, as guide and mentor to those of other related caring professions, e.g. doctors, until they have acquired experience and expertise. It is a difficult role, as it often goes unappreciated and unrecognized. It can lead to conflict situations, especially if there are obvious omissions, and sometimes doubtful practices. Each nurse has to decide to what extent she can condone doubtful professional practice in others, when it is likely to have an adverse effect on her clientele, and when senior members of the team or management have to be alerted to possible, dangerous shortfalls. Some of the qualities required of nurses in contentious situations are assertiveness, not aggressiveness, tact, diplomacy, a sound knowledge base on which to form judgements or opinions and the political skills to formulate recommendations and statements in an acceptable manner.

It is questionable whether the school nurse should act as chaperone for a whole session of medical examinations, though she may opt to do so in instances where the outcomes are crucial, for example in cases of suspected child abuse. It is a strange situation which has become accepted practice, that male doctors require chaperoning, whereas female doctors are usually left alone with their client or patient. The nurse or doctor may also feel that an experienced person's presence is helpful, for example, if the young person is potentially violent or when the parents are overtly aggressive. Young children may welcome the presence of the nurse as a familiar figure, especially if their own parents cannot be present, and they do not know the medical officer, or are frightened of being examined. The ideal situation is when parents are invited and accept the invitation to be present at their child's examination, and when doctor and nurse agree prior to any session the aspects to be especially explored, as well as discussing the outcomes afterwards.

The nurse's major functions during medical examinations are: to provide health education on an individual basis as appropriate to those children attending; to complete or repeat any assessment procedures which are outstanding and needed as background to the efficient examination of the child; to discuss matters of relevance with those parents who are attending and waiting; and sometimes to reassure the parents and child and explain to them what is about to occur, why is has been found necessary or helpful, and often to interpret what has actually happened in the medical room. The nurse may also be responsible for ensuring that the appropriate equipment is available so that examinations can be carried out, to ascertain that prophylactic materials, such as vaccines, are obtained, noting their batch numbers and expiry dates, and generally prepare for the smooth running of the session. She would have prepared and informed the school that such a session was taking place, and decided which children would be required to attend. Preferably, she will have drafted a time schedule so that the teachers can indicate where children are to be found, and avoid waste of time and effort. The schedule can be used for children to be sent to the medical room; if children have to be taken from classes, the nurse should have assistance to do so. It is a clerical task to send out the invitations to attend for medical examinations and the nurse should be able to inform the person responsible for performing this task of the children and parents to be invited, and of the number who can be seen at any one session. The last is often not made clear, and some clerical officers invite more children than can be thoroughly examined – only the medical or educational team members can guesstimate that there are reasons which may protract a session and limit numbers. Computerized systems make the process easier, and can produce the schedule at the same time as the invitations, as well as notifying any deviance from established procedures or any omissions. The nurse will need to know what computer system is in operation and what she requires this system to do for her, she should then be able to leave the computer experts to produce the goods.

SPECIFIC HYGIENE SURVEYS

Hygiene surveys have formed part of the nurse's role as long as there have been school nurses. They have concentrated on the elimination of infestations with a remarkable lack of success. Over the past few years, there has been much debate about whether routine surveys are cost-effective, whether they are necessary and whether general hygiene education could achieve more, and more quickly than surveys. It seems clear that the nurse's role in eliminating infestations is limited, and that the responsibility rests with parents and public. The nurse should concentrate on informing and teaching about 'pests', their lifestyle and how to deal with them. It is also clear that teachers' expectations are at variance with the informed opinion of health professionals. Some health authorities have defined policies about hygiene surveys, others are inclined to 'play it by ear'. Whatever the policy or practice, each nurse must be familiar with the details of infestations, the sight, sound and smell of vermin, the life-cycle of such creatures, and the most effective means of extermination. She must be able to act, inform and demonstrate how to act. If and when such surveys are carried out, they should not concentrate on the physical presence of the suspected infestation agent, but seek the sources, and use the session for generalized debate on health matters. It is sad, and not commensurate with present-day professionalism, if children only associate the school nurse with head inspection – it has taken a long time for the image of the 'nit-nurse' to fade.

Hygiene surveys on a broader basis can be useful, especially among older children who are expected to provide self-care. They often highlight lack of knowledge among children or lack of facilities, and they can uncover such matters as solvent or drug abuse. The signs of abuse, such as, for example, sores around the mouth and nose, insipient catarrh, eye-pupil size, needle marks or excessive irritability, can become more evident when a group is seen together, than when individuals are seen alone; allowance should always be made for possible personal idiosyncracies.

PROPHYLACTIC MEASURES

Nurses will be involved in preparing for or participating in sessions providing immunizations and vaccinations. It has already been indicated in Chapter 5 that nurses do not have direct responsibility for 'giving' prophylaxis, but may have delegated responsibility. The actuality of any prophylactic programme changes repeatedly as new products become available and as knowledge about effectiveness or side-effects changes. The nurse therefore has to be familiar with the practice and programmes proposed at national and local levels, with the products and dosages recommended for use. She must also know about research findings indicating the optimum age for effectiveness and about the possible hazards during administration, as well as any side-effects. She has to know how to deal with reactions to the substances; which reactions can be contained and are self-limiting, and which require immediate treatment and referral. Many nurses will be approached by children, parents or teachers who are preparing for visits abroad, and will wish to know the measures required or advisable for countries to be visited. It would be unlikely that any individual nurse could know all the measures available at any one time, but she should know where to find the most up-to-date information, such as government guidelines or emigration and visa conditions, and where enquirers can obtain these measures in any locality. In many instances, general medical practitioners are able to obtain the required substances, but it is more likely that these are stored and provided at a central point.

Currently, all children should be protected against: diphtheria; tetanus; and poliomyelitis. Additionally, all girls should be offered protection against rubella (German measles). All children are also offered protection against whooping cough; and, until recently, all children were also offered protection against smallpox, but this is no longer true in all parts of the country. All children who intend to travel abroad should be offered this prophylactic measure.

All children are offered a test (Heaf or Mantoux) for resistance to infection by tuberculosis; those found not to be immune are offered a prophylactic measure (BCG). In some parts of the country the incidence of tuberculosis and therefore the chance of infection was considered to be so low that this procedure was not considered cost-effective. In other parts of the country, such as some inner city areas, the incidence is high and notification of new infections has escalated to such an extent that this measure is now, or rather once again, offered pre-school and often post-natally; so the test for maintenance of resistance (antibodies) at approximately 14 years of age is crucial.

Other prophylactic measures include protection against measles, yellow fever, malaria and sleeping sickness. Some of these are provided at the recommendation of the World Health Organization when visiting or working in certain countries, because despite WHO's extensive programmes for eradication of diseases, success is slow, and some countries make entry conditional upon immunization of particular kinds. Of the short list given above, measles is the most surprising. In the UK and most Western countries, measles is a nuisance but generally not a dangerous condition. In some countries measles is extremely virulent and can be a killer disease.

All prophylactic substances given routinely are preventive measures for potentially lethal or crippling diseases, and only high uptake levels, and thereby resistance within the population, can ensure that deaths and disasters do not result. The disease-causing organisms have not been totally eliminated; they continue to be endemic in their places of origin, and any lack of vigilance can lead to serious outbreaks of the disease.

Nurses have a special role in persuading parents and children to consent to receive prophylaxis, in explaining the dangers and procedures and in reassuring about the minimal discomfort which might be experienced. They are likely to be involved closely with 'defaulters', or those who are willing to accept one 'dose', but not the whole measure of three or four, and who expect effectiveness to be complete despite incompleteness of series or excessive exposure. They may also have to explain that immunity has a limited time-span, variable with each disease and its prophylactic measure, and that repetition for some people is essential to provide protection. The prophylactic status of nurses and doctors, i.e. those who provide the measures, may also be questioned, and merits consideration.

CLINIC SESSIONS

Some nurses have provided clinic facilities in past years, and some continue to do so. These have generally been for the treatment of minor ailments, including the continuing treatment of cuts, bruises, verrucas, cold sores and a range of annoying and distressing manifestations of growing-up, such as skin conditions of adolescence. It is questionable whether such clinic sessions should continue or whether the need for them has been obviated. If nurses have regular contact sessions in school settings, they can advise on all of these matters without the need to use special premises and committing additional and scarce time. Some school nurses may provide input at specialist clinics, e.g. child guidance, and some may be additionally qualified to provide coverage of family planning and other clinics. In general, it would seem that clinic work is the least onerous of the nurse's tasks, and any commitment to it should be carefully evaluated.

ORGANIZATION OF WORK

Professional practice implies that the work to be accomplished has to be organized in a way which facilitates successful outcomes. In some instances, such as nursing within a hospital environment, organization has to be on a broad span, incorporating all those dealing with a group of patients, within a ward or department and ensuring that the skills mix available is appropriate and adequate for all occasions. The individual therefore must subsume the organization of their own work to the greater number.

Within community settings, including school nursing, each individual carries a caseload for which she is responsible and has to organize the workload to encompass as much as possible in each hour, each day, each week and throughout each year. There continues to be a need for taking account of others' input or responsibilities in relation to the case/workload, and for the skills mix required to best serve the population. Because no one works in isolation there has to be some broad organization for the work, such as coverage of leave of all kinds, coverage of fixed sessions, such as medical examinations and clinics, and assurance that the priorities within each case/workload are met. This part of the organization of work is usually the responsibility of 'management', but should closely involve each practitioner. It also relates to accountability which has been discussed in previous chapters.

Definitions of case and workload are sometimes confusing, and often misinterpreted. Generally speaking, *caseload* means the total population to be served, e.g. the number of schools, their pupils, parents and teachers for which a nurse carries responsibility, and encompasses those within the population to whom one may not have access or who may not accept services or advice; *workload* means that proportion of the population actually served, the sessions held, the assessments carried out and the health teaching provided. Official definitions are scarce; Appendix D is an adaptation of the definition given by the English National Board for Nurses, Midwives and Health Visitors for fieldwork teachers.

Each nurse or health visitor within the community has to organize her own work within the parameters of the case/workload and job specification. In the first instance, this entails a precise analysis of the content of both; not only population figures, but also the composition, age and social structure, defined health needs, perceived health care needs, other services available and the time and resources which can be channelled. Second, and based on this analysis, the nurse must decide those aspects of the load which require a regular, routine approach, those which are urgent and form priorities and those which can be dealt with safely at later stages. The decision must allow flexibility to include referrals or newly arising matters and crises. Among the latter may be coverage for colleagues who are absent, sudden epidemics or changes in policy which require a concerted approach about a particular health care provision.

Essential to successful organization is regular review, so that changes in every facet can be accommodated and utilized for the benefit of nurses and their clientele.

Third, each nurse will have to evolve a system of day-to-day organization which enables her to practice effectively, and which can be clearly understood by others, especially managers and colleagues. Some of the detailed organization may be idiosyncratic, but usually it involves the use of planning charts or calenders, diaries and summaries of completed work. The method should make use of all available resources and be modified to incorporate anything which may ease the load, and makes use of new materials and developments. It is often wise to set aside a few minutes every month to consider the materials available which will assist in effective organization; only well-considered requests for their supply are likely to be acceded to.

It would appear that one of the most difficult organizational aspects is the management of one's time. Within educational and other community settings it is not always possible to allocate time precisely, as there are repeated unknown factors such as traffic jams, self-referrals, sudden crisis and sudden severe stresses, as well as unspecified numbers of people to be cared for and communicated with, all of which require adjustments to work which can be accomplished at any given time. However, it is possible and necessary to estimate the time spent on each activity, the time it may take to travel between sites and appointments, and allow spaces which can be used to deal with the unexpected or deal with 'routine' matters, which may otherwise slip too far to the end of the list of priorities. It is also essential to reassess priorities at regular intervals, because they may change and to ensure that routine elements do not get omitted or forgotten.

The organization of records, of required statistical returns, of work diaries and of nursing, medical or treatment rooms are the most obvious, practical and therefore easiest of all aspects of organization. As they appear to be so easy and based on common sense, they are often given too little attention. Well-organized systems for each can save time and trouble.

Nurses do not usually excel at delegating work. Successful delegation of some tasks, effective supervision and guidance of ancillary staff, co-operation with voluntary helpers and co-ordination of efforts by all members of a team, can make organization of work a pleasure instead of a chore, and can lead to changes in the workload which allow an enhanced service to all those within the caseload.

Work organization is not a static entity, and needs review and revision at regular intervals. Any nurse working in the community has to be able to demonstrate that she can organize and manage herself, the time and resources available, her case/workload and the parameters surrounding these. There are times and situations, such as personal ill-health or excessive tiredness, when organization becomes difficult. Each nurse has to assess, or rely on the guidance of her peers, the point at which she needs to seek advice and help with either the management of her caseload or the organization of her workload. Some health authorities require copies of a proposed work-schedule, i.e. the statement of intent to be at particular sites or addresses with approximate timings, to be submitted to a central point or deposited at an agreed venue, daily or weekly. Generally, although this is one management tool, this is a safety measure, aimed at the protection of staff in potentially violent settings.

OBSERVATION VISITS

During the course in school nursing opportunity is usually provided to observe some special or alternate practice. This may be important for those who are inexperienced; it is equally important for those who have practiced in relative isolation for some time and who may be advantaged by noting how others achieve the same or similar objectives. Such observation visits can only be valuable if there is preparation for them, i.e. clear ideas regarding the possible advantages to be gained, the questions to be asked and the rationale for each visit. It is essential that the host is also prepared to demonstrate, explain and answer the questions posed, and that sufficient forward planning occurs for each visit to be non-intrusive and non-disruptive. The most beneficial aspect of such visits is the sharing of information and impressions afterwards, i.e. the vocalizing and internalizing of the new skills and knowledge. It is likely that in any short course observation visits are kept to a minimum, but this should not prevent the same process occurring after qualification. The organization of work may include the observation of others' practice, in order to enhance each other's knowledge and skills, and to learn new methods and ideas.

ASSESSING PROFESSIONAL COMPETENCE

At the end of a course leading to recording of the qualification, such as a course in school nursing, each student will be assessed regarding her competence to practice (HMSO, 1983). The course will only be successfully completed, and recommendation for recording made, if this assessment proves positive. Since 1979, when courses were first provided, various means of assessing competence have been tried. Initially, there had to be reliance on assessors whose experience of school nursing was variable, but who were responsible for the school-aged population within a patch or district. These could be nursing officers or health visitors. Gradually, it has become possible for qualified and experienced school nurses to take on the role of assessor. Additionally, more nursing officers or senior nurses have been appointed to positions of responsibility for child and school health. In all training institutions providing courses in school nursing, assessors receive some form of induction to assessment; in many they are invited to attend short courses specifically to learn the skills required. Assessment of competence for professional practice is not an easy matter. The assessor has to ensure that a minimum standard, and hopefully skills beyond this minimum, is achieved, that experienced and inexperienced students can demonstrate the same level of basic skills, and that all of those assessed are safe to practice without constant supervision. The skills incorporate those acquired during nursing, and those required to practice in educational settings. The assessor also has the onerous task of accounting to an examination board, and possibly being required to explain and justify her recommendation. The greatest dilemma is encountered when assessment demonstrates insufficiency, and when this pertains to an existing employee, possibly a person who has apparently practiced for some time before undertaking the course. Statutory Instrument 873 (HMSO, 1983) states the competences required of nurses, midwives and health visitors on completion of training; the competences required of other post-registration courses are enshrined in their syllabi.

Assessment of competence is not only a matter of obtaining a qualification, but continues throughout professional practice. Employers are responsible for ascertaining that people appointed to posts which require particular skills are competent, as well as qualified on paper, and that these competences are maintained and extended. Employees are responsible to ensure that they maintain their basic competences, that they update them and that they acquire new ones commensurate with changes and developments in the practical situation. The policy of establishing a 'live' register formulated by the UKCC and coming into operation in 1987, is one step underpinning this; it will require proof of competence after any break in 'active service' in the foreseeable future, and proof of competence at all times in the more distant future.

Each professional practitioner also has a responsibility to assist entrants to the profession, and to help those newly qualified and inexperienced to acquire the relevant skills, knowledge and attitudes, i.e. to take on a teaching role. Part of this consists of the presentation of self as a role model; partly it means being able and willing to demonstrate and explain practice; and finally it means being willing to exchange opinions and ideas and learn from each other. Newcomers to any profession are attracted by the people within it and their willingness to welcome them; they bring new ideas and stimulation to established professionals. The mixture provides a fertile environment for success.

SUMMARY

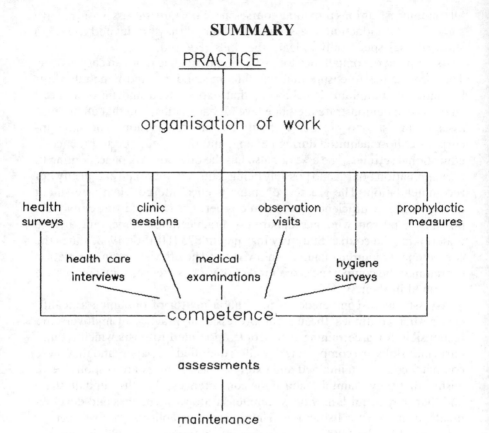

PRACTICE

organisation of work

health surveys	clinic sessions	observation visits	prophylactic measures

health care interviews medical examinations hygiene surveys

competence

assessments

maintenance

REFERENCES

DHSS (1978) *Assessment Schedule*, DHSS, London.

HMSO (1983) *Statutory Instrument 873*, HMSO, London.

Nash, W. (1985) *Health at School*, Heinemann, London.

National Boards for Nursing, Midwifery and Health Visiting for England, Wales, Scotland and Northern Ireland (1985) *Syllabus for a Course in School Nursing*, ENBX, London.

9
PROFESSIONAL DEVELOPMENT

Professional development consists of many facets and phases. One phase is the completion of initial training, providing general identification with a large professional group and the legality of actually being a nurse. Then there is usually the phase of consolidation of nursing knowledge and practice through experience. The period of consolidation can be very variable, depending partly on the chronological age of the person, but to a greater extent on the development of special interests, maturity of outlook and personal experiences which may enhance or inhibit professionalism.

The next important phase is normally reached when the person is ready emotionally, professionally and physically or geographically to proceed to post-registration education and training. It used to be the norm for nurses to acquire a second qualification, most often midwifery (SCM) or a combination of SRN/RMN or SRN/RSCN, though any permutation of about 45 was possible. Most nurses and employers now recognize that the acquisition of qualifications is not a satisfactory guide to expertise and competence; they look for relevant qualifications, that is education and training, which enhance the ability to perform in different settings, and which are most likely to meet the needs of a job specification. This is reflected in changed patterns of training courses at post-registration levels; some have been extended, a few have disappeared (for example, training to be a registered fever nurse), and new entities have developed, for example, courses on children with special needs. There has also been differentiation between those qualifications which are an *absolute* pre-condition for obtaining appointments, i.e. for practice, such as becoming a Registered General

Nurse (RGN), a Registered Midwife (RM) or a Registered Health Visitor (RHV); those which *are required* for obtaining appointments, i.e. which are mandatory for practice but are recordable and not registrable, such as, for example, becoming a District Nurse, a Lecturer in Health Visting, a Nurse Teacher or a Fieldwork or Practical Work Teacher; and those which are recordable as a *highly recommended* and desirable qualifications for practice, such as successful completion of the Course in School Nursing or the course in intensive care nursing. There are also a range of courses which deal with specialisms within nursing and which employers may make a condition of appointment (Nurses, Midwives and Health Visitors Act, 1979; UKCC, 1983–1986; National Board guide to post-registration courses, 1986).

No course of preparation can nowadays enable the practitioner to remain competent throughout professional life, and a range of refresher, updating, in-service and development courses are available. Access to these courses, as well as uptake, is very variable, but generally employers have accepted the need for all staff to participate at regular intervals. In general, staff working in community settings, including educational ones, have been more aware of the need to keep abreast of developments, perhaps because the scenario within the community is a constantly shifting one, whereas staff in more sheltered settings, such as some hospitals, have not been as responsive to this need. It is well worth reiterating that professional updating and development are a shared responsibility between practitioner and manager or employer; both have to define and agree educational needs, and there has to be negotiated agreement regarding the part played and provision made by either and both.

Some health authority employers have difficulties in matching the educational needs of their staff, even when these have been clearly identified, with the exigencies of the service and allocation of resources, the latter including time for study, relief from some duties and financial support. In recent years resource allocation for continuing education has become more widespread, in parallel with the recognition that in the long-term resources are actually saved, if staff are enabled to carry out their functions competently, make appropriate use of modern techniques and can be held responsible for their professional actions. Some authorities have, very practically, found that competent staff provide an unparalleled reservoir of resources which had previously remained untapped, and that competence can lead to savings in time, repetition, legal costs (because there is less likelihood of things going wrong), and not least that competent practitioners achieve more job satisfaction, leading to reduced staff turnover and wastage.

This forms the base-line for any professional development, though it has been applied to nursing. On the whole, nurses have been slow to recognize the importance and relevance of this area, though they form one of the largest occupational groups in the country. Could the underlying reason be that until relatively recently nursing was predominantly a female occupation, and that despite the emergence of males within the profession as a strong and ambitious force, the general public and the 'powers that be' still regard nursing as a female, and therefore secondary, profession? There are, of course, other important aspects to professional development, some of which are discussed below.

CAREER STRUCTURE

Nursing has been based historically and (unfortunately) practically on a hierarchical system.

Matron
Deputy Matron and/or departmental heads
Sister (Health Visitor, District Nurse, some School Nurses)
Other Qualified Nurses
Final Year Student Nurses
Skivvies

This perception is slow to dissipate. The present management structure, for both hospital and community, is still rooted in the past, though more variations on themes are both possible and found in practice. From 1974 until 1984 the nursing hierarchy could be seen as follows (NHS Reorganization Act, 1973):

Regional Nursing Officer + Staff posts
District Nursing Officer + Staff posts
Divisional Nursing Officer + Staff posts
Senior Nursing Officer(s)
Nursing Officer(s)
Other Qualified Staff
Learner nurses (2nd and 3rd year)
Skivvies

Both of these patterns, with the exception of regional and district levels, were repeated for most specialities within nursing. Since 1984 the management structure, while still hierarchical, does not require nurses to be accountable to nurses, but may have many variations on the theme of management (NHS Reorganization Act, 1982). The posts listed below, except the 'lower' ones, are open for competition by anyone who can demonstrate to the selectors that they may be able to 'manage' the job, and that they consider themselves to be knowledgeable and skilful at this. It is regrettable that insufficient nurses appear, as yet, to be sufficiently competitive to have been successful in obtaining senior management posts, nor have they been sufficiently assertive to demonstrate their commitment to the future in acceptable terms.

It is also of note that each reorganizational change has purported to aim at reductions in management levels, and to alleviate existing duplications or confusions. One of the imperatives of the future is that nurses become expert in all the arenas of management, skilled in budget control, more than familiar with manpower planning and resource allocation, and above all actively and energetically competitive with others. Any certainty that qualification plus experience will lead to promotion no longer exists, nor is the ability to perform the job sufficient guarantee of advancement. The present structure varies for the 196 districts within the 14 health regions which form the NHS, but can be summarized as follows:

Regional Team:
with someone, usually a nurse, responsible for 'quality control'.
District General Manager:
with nursing advisory facilities
as well as specialist advice and staff posts in some instances
(at present approximately 24 per cent of District General Managers
hold nursing qualifications).
Unit General Managers:
the number of these varies
according to the number of units within a district
(at present approximately 58 per cent of Unit General Managers
hold nursing qualifications).
Staff posts:
at district and/or unit levels,
such as child health/local authority liaison
(usually a nurse).
Senior Nurses:
subjected to a vast variety of titles
with and without caseloads,
management roles, roles as assessors of practice, etc.
Qualified staff:
with various responsibilities, including management roles
at local levels.

Learners:
especially student nurses beyond the introductory block.
Skivvies.

The actual number of nurses in positions of responsibility within management structures which rose in and after 1974, became a strong and competent force by 1982; it has diminished considerably since 1983/4 (NHS Reorganization Act, 1982). The question should be asked 'To whom did the strength pose a threat?'. During the decade of success there were people specially designated and qualified as managers of school nursing in approximately 50 per cent of districts and 65 per cent of divisions.

School nurses should be part of the move to regain and strengthen the teams of nurse managers, and the acquisition of recognizable management skills should become part of future professional development.

The career structure and career development of school nurses is therefore largely uncertain, with the gains of the last decade where some nurse managers became directly responsible for school nursing services being jeopardized, like many other senior nursing posts. School nurses will have to negotiate, and prepare themselves for competition, to gain management posts at any level of the nursing structure.

Alternatively, school nurses can become clinical nurse specialists, experts in the field of school health, and recognized as such by the role they undertake *vis-à-vis* their colleagues and entrants or newcomers to the profession. They can become the designated nurse of the health authority in matters relating to the assessment of children, or the nurse responsible for child health services. The latter spans children of pre-school and school age, and will therefore require additional expertise in the care and management of infants and young children, and additional knowledge related to child abuse and child-related legislation, as well as detailed awareness of local authority services and the establishment of relationships with other agencies.

The third strand of career progression is linked to teaching, either at grass-roots level, as supervisor and mentor to post-registration, and possibly general nurse learners, or at college bases. This requires a commitment to academic as well as professional development, something which will be relatively new to this professional group, but of which many of its members are more than capable.

The fourth strand is still unknown, but it consists of being opportunistic in utilizing all available opportunities for development and study, and creating new ones. The certainty of further changes inside and outside of the health service may give rise to a range of chances for career development.

The fifth strand already exists, but is grossly under-utilized by all nurses, namely, to participate actively in professional activities at local and national levels. It would be nice to look forward to the day when representation of school nurses on public bodies, health authorities, local authorities, boards of governors, local councils and in Parliament became the norm rather than the exception. There are a number of school nurses who play an active part in public life, either as members of organizations, professional or voluntary, or as partners to their husbands. It would be even more exciting to have school nurses in official capacities, elected in their own right, possibly accompanied by husband or child as appendage. One arena where school nurses should be very active, both as professionals and as citizens, is in the field of consumer protection.

ACADEMIC DEVELOPMENT

Currently, there are no school nurses qualified, i.e. recorded, to act as nurse teachers, and therefore none who can apply for posts as course leaders to courses in school nursing. All such leadership roles are currently taken by Lecturers in Health Visiting; professional development may actively seek to change this situation.

There are usually two routes which can lead to qualification as a teacher. One is to obtain graduate status, and supplement this with specific teaching courses; the other is to be seconded for recognized training as a nurse or technical teacher at approved centres or institutions. Some school nurses have already taken the first step in this direction. They have obtained degrees or are undertaking degree studies; others have taken teaching qualifications. The unfortunate reality of the latter is that few or none of those school nurses currently holding teaching qualifications have followed courses at approved levels or approved institutions and they can therefore not be recorded as holding this qualification.

Many school nurses are now undertaking the supervision of entrants to their profession, and performing the role of assessors of practice. Most institutions providing courses for school nurses have held induction courses into this role. A few have admitted school nurses into their course for Assessors of Supervized Practice, and most recently the facility has been created for school nurses to join general nurses in Practice Teaching courses. It yet remains for this development to receive official recognition.

Academic development does not have to depend on access to and availability of courses in the vicinity. Organizations such as the Open University and Open Tech (started in Spring 1987) are providing opportunities for everybody. It requires considerable self-discipline to follow a programme of study in one's own time, at one's own home and, within limits, at one's own pace. The discipline and the challenge concentrates the mind wonderfully. Some people find this preferable to making commitments for being in a given place at a given time. Distance-learning opportunities are increasing rapidly; materials are being developed by various institutions and organizations, for example, at the distance learning resources unit of the Polytechnic of the South Bank, London, and Mersey Health Authority's training package (MRHA, 1986). The mass media, especially television, can provide another means of continuing education, but before this can be used successfully, critical faculties require active development.

It should be mentioned, though it is likely to be relevant for a few people only, that there is no age limit on obtaining GCE O and A level qualifications. Most local adult education institutes, some correspondence courses and some schools make these basic studies available to all-comers. It is also possible to enter for GCE examinations without having followed any structured course, provided that the examination regulations do not require evidence of specified practical work.

Correspondence courses are available from a range of institutions for a range of subjects and leading to a range of qualifications. Careful selection is necessary, but it does demonstrate that there are opportunities for everybody.

The cost of study varies from relatively nominal amounts at local adult education centres to £100 and more at the Open University, and very variable amounts for other courses. It is not always easy or possible to obtain financial support for such studies, but there are some avenues available (Daniels, revised biennially).

Development should include a broadening of perspectives, an increase in knowledge, and the gaining of new knowledge. There is considerable debate whether new knowledge should be job-specific or whether learning of any subject can enhance professional performance. It seems probable that most newly acquired knowledge, as well as extended information and its use, of any subject leads to a reconsideration of one's practice and thereby enhances performance and skills; most importantly it affects attitudes, usually in a positive direction. It is certain that continued learning leads to receptive minds which will be able to analyse situations, act in a fashion based on a range of data, be pro-active and innovative in their approach to any job, but especially in their consideration of health needs and community activity, and will be enabled to share this increasing wisdom with colleagues and others.

PERSONAL DEVELOPMENT

No professional development can be complete without the individual developing on personal levels. It is impossible to be specific about the way any person should enhance or change their personality, but it seems appropriate for the practice of school nursing that such changes should incorporate contact with a range of people and professions, an understanding of the social contexts which may affect people, and an awareness of changes which are happening outside the nursing ambit, e.g. unemployment, economic strategies, demographic or technological changes which affect daily living, and political influences at local and national levels. The development of effective communication skills, an essential for any school nurse, can be enhanced by using such skills in a private capacity. Other interpersonal skills needed for nursing practice can become a matter of relative ease if the nurse is able to form and maintain personal relationships in her private capacity. It has been clearly shown, by sickness absence records and performance reviews, that personal problems, especially interpersonal problems, can affect professional functions (Office of Health Economics, 1981, 1982, 1983).

Most people benefit and therefore perform better professionally if they maintain a range of interests outside their working life. It does not appear to matter whether these interests are solitary or social, creative or physically active, intellectual or intensely practical; the important feature appears to be that they prevent the person from becoming a 'workaholic', which can be a rather dismal addiction, and in the long term affects not only the person, but also those with whom he or she associates personally and professionally.

Many people will seek to actively change some aspects of their personality. In some instances this may be desirable, but no research has proven whether it is successful or beneficial, or whether it just leads to the emergence of other equally problematic personality traits. There are a few traits which are basic requirements of professionalism, such as reliability, honesty and absence of criminal tendencies.

ROLE PROGRESSION

Career and personal development have now been considered, but there is another important factor related to professional practice, namely role progression, or development within and of one's role in the chosen field of work. On completion of training or on entering a new post, the post-holder is likely to have a range of skills and knowledge which allows the fulfilment of the job specification. Often there will be a period when the person adapts to a new professional environment, a new clientele and the specified parameters of the role. This period should be limited, but in reality lasts from a few weeks to too many years. Adaptation should be followed by competence and confidence in carrying out the role and its functions. Some people are content to maintain this as a status quo, but it can be argued that maintenance of such a state is in fact regression. Each person needs stimuli to continue at optimum capacity, and one very effective stimulus can be to consider ways and means to develop the given role. No professional role should ever be static, though dynamism does have inherent stresses, and no professional need be circumscribed by the parameters of the role as indicated in a job specification. The latter usually states the requirements expected by an employer, it is part of professional practice to fulfil those requirements by the most appropriate means at one's disposal, and change those means when professional judgement indicates such change. Additionally, some aspects of the role become repetitive; the practitioner gets used to them. There are two possible sequals: either practice becomes superficial and slipshod, an undesirable outcome, or practice develops either in parts or as a whole and thereby role progression is created. Most roles have sufficient leeway to allow substantial developments and progression; some have to be negotiated with colleagues and others, others have to be documented and proven to be workable and applicable.

There is considerable reluctance among some practitioners to move beyond the accepted, traditional patterns. They feel uneasy in case they are not seen to be successful, or in case they have to experiment in order to find the best way forward. It is usual for one person, or a small group of people, to act as pioneers – *when*, and not *if*, they share their experiences with others, they usually find measures of support as well as suspicion. The most disheartening, and at the same time the most challenging and positive, element is that one person's role progression in time becomes established practice and the whole cycle has to commence again. Role progression implies self- or peer evaluation at regular intervals, and a commitment to enhance and perfect practice. It also implies that the ideas and ideals of the espoused profession, in this instance the promotion of positive health in the school-aged population, the prevention and containment of disease and handicap, and education towards healthy lifestyles, behaviours and attitudes, are kept under constant review. The rewards are usually intrinsic rather than materialistic, and the motivating force has to emanate from internal strengths.

Some people find that contact with students, newcomers to the profession, acts as an additional stimulus. Achievement of progression puts the person on many occasions in the position of catalyst *vis-à-vis* other practitioners, and can lead to career opportunities and progression. Unfortunately, the latter then requires the same process to be repeated in the new role, and by other practitioners. Career progression can only affect role progression if the person acts as a stimulant to others in the new role.

DEVELOPING A PROFESSIONAL IDENTITY

Nursing has been regarded as a 'minor' profession, despite the vast numbers employed within it. This is partly due to the predominance of females within the profession, and therefore the chauvinistic attitudes displayed towards it, partly due to the medical domination which has until recently been accepted by so many, and partly due to the low wage and thereby status accorded to nursing. The latter is a remnant of the Nightingale legacy, which made nurses out of 'educated young ladies' and which led to an inculcation of subservience during nurse training. It also relates to the use of learners as the majority of the workforce. It is only relatively recently that nursing has acquired a strong voice and become organized into representative groups. Nursing has also suffered by the fact that there were and are many splinter and specialist groups within it. The last decade has seen a strengthening of the various groups, and a realization that they have to be strong on two levels: first, their speciality or special interest and, second, the profession as a whole.

School nursing has been no exception. The last decade has seen the emergence of local school nurses' groups and then the affiliation of many groups and individuals to a central core – the Amalgamated School Nurses, Association (ASNA) – so that the voice could become unanimous and strong.

In parallel, the school nurses' groups, which have for many years been a nominal part of larger organizations, such as the Health Visitors Association (HVA) or the Royal College of Nursing (RCN), have gained renewed strengths and found means of representing their members at many levels, making their opinions known and voices heard. This has had at least two far-reaching and profound effects: first, it has made school nursing become recognized as an entity and has led to the incorporation of the group's views into debates and discussions of policy issues, the seeking of their comments before decisions affecting them have been reached and respect for any views expressed; second, it has led to school nurses having a recognizable identity and being proud of this. All the indicators show that this process will continue and that the school nurse identity will develop into a force to be reckoned with.

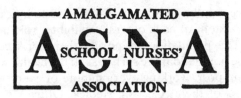

SCHOOL NURSES GROUP

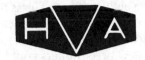

SCHOOL NURSE FORUM

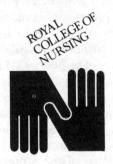

The situation is, of course, more complex than stated above. Professional identity is not acquired easily, either individually or as a group. There has to be proven competence in practice, the recognition of need as useful employees, and the acceptance of the position by the community and society in general. School nurses suffered for many years from 'a bad press', or a very weak image. It has taken time and considerable effort to overcome the 'head inspector' or 'nit-nurse' perspective held and perpetuated by society. Individual nurses in their educational settings have been accorded respect and trust, but by the diffuse nature of their past work it has not always been possible for them to be integrated sufficiently into the primary health care or educational teams for their true value to be appreciated.

The emergence of a professional identity among a 'new' group can present a threat to established groups. Occasionally, the increase in competence and confidence is matched with increases in resentment, jealousy and even active 'blockage' or defence tactics by others. School nurses and health visitors are notorious for their animosity to each other, though many work together very successfully. This appears to be due to lack of recognition on both sides of the extent of each others' capability, role and functions and case/workload. The populations requiring their services and the health needs within these populations are such that all the health visitors and school nurses currently in post, working every minute of every working day, still could not meet all of them. Clinical Medical Officers have occasionally, despite the protection of their medicalism, felt very insecure because the school nurse is the expert in school health, and usually knows the range of circumstances relating to the children seen. This is becoming more acute, as the medical officers' role is threatened by other factors, mainly political and economic. Still others bring preconceived notions to their relationships with school nurses; general medical practitioners could be one example, and it takes time and persuasion to change attitudes.

It has already been mentioned that the identity or image of the school nurse has suffered because the profession is predominantly female. Not only are women regarded – still – by many as second-class citizens, and treated accordingly, but many women, including school nurses, accept this position unquestioningly. The emergence of professional identity has been in tandem with women's changed role, especially the refusal to be treated as second-raters. At long last women, again including school nurses, are recognizing their own worth, and acting accordingly, not least by expecting others to accord them respect and recognition. Occasionally, there is still evidence that some school nurses undervalue themselves; the identity crisis will not be fully overcome until each member of the profession values herself as she would wish to be seen by others.

This change in stance is not easy, indeed it is often difficult for a woman to combine her professional role with her traditional roles of wife, mother, housekeeper, maid of all work and informal carer of relatives of all ages. Adjustments usually have to be made; the scanty evidence available suggests that a partnership approach to traditional roles, especially marriage, and a more pragmatic approach to other roles strengthens and eases, through diminution of guilt feelings, the professional identity. There is some, though unproven, evidence that children benefit by a mother's broader development, and that they respect and admire the professional identity of a parent.

SUMMARY

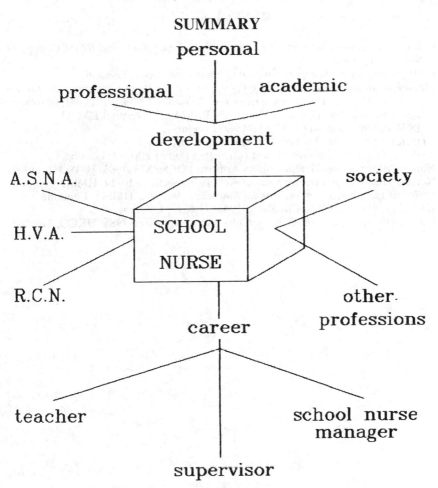

USEFUL ADDRESSES

Amalgamated School Nurses' Association (ASNA). Chairperson: M. Dams, 8
Western Road, Henley-on-Thames, Oxon.
Distance Learning Resources Unit, Polytechnic of the South Bank, London E1.
Health Visitors Association (HVA) – School Nurses Group, Chairperson: L. Pratt,
c/o HVA, 50 Southwark Street, London E1.
Open University, Department of Health and Social Welfare, Walton Hall, Milton
Keynes MK7 6AA.
Royal College of Nursing, School Nurses Forum, c/o Cavendish Square, London
W1.

REFERENCES

Daniels, N. (revised biennially) *Guide to Grants and Bursaries*, Royal College of Nursing, London.

ENB (annually) *Post-registration course handbook*, ENB, London.

Mersey Regional Health Authority (1986) *Person to Person – Putting the Service Back into Health – The Effective Customer Relations Training Package*, in association with NHSTA, Hamilton House, 24 Pall Mall, Liverpool L3 6AL.

NHS Reorganization Act (1973) HMSO, London.

NHS Reorganization Act (1982) HMSO, London.

NHS Management Enquiry Report (Griffiths) (1983) HMSO, London.

Nurses, Midwives and Health Visitors Approval Order 873 (1983) HMSO, London.

Nurses, Midwives and Health Visitors Act (1979) Sections 10–14, HMSO, London.

Office of Health Economics, *Annual Statistical Analysis*, HMSO, London.

UKCC (1983) Reg/83/00, Circulated 1983, UKCC, London.

UKCC (1986) PS & D/86/02, paragraphs 2 & 3, circulated 1986, UKCC, London.

10
IMAGES OF SCHOOL NURSING

Perception and the image of school nursing and school nurses have been mentioned several times in this book. It is very important to realize that the image held by oneself and others is a vital component of the present situation. This includes role and functions, esteem or respect and self-respect, the possibilities for a realistic career and management structure, and any form of career development. It is even more vital when considering possibilities for the future, as discussed in Chapter 12. Perceptions do not always match reality, but are usually an amalgam of preconceived notions, information and misinformation, desired or hoped-for truths, ideals and a modicum of fact. Images persist through time, when the mixture has changed in many ways. They are often a comfortable way of coping, not being threatened by change and not acknowledging what effect one change may have on others; nor does it require the effort of changing one's ideas. Very often perceptions and images are unacknowledged, subconscious and therefore very hard to determine and amend. Perceptions and images will always remain somewhat of a dilemma, as it remains difficult to define what constitutes a professional, e.g. what makes a school nurse, and what should make 'such a person'. This chapter is included to raise awareness and stimulate debate, though it does not exhaust the subject.

HISTORICAL LEGACY

Many people, clients and colleagues from nursing and other disciplines hold the image of the school nurse as it was some two or more decades ago. At that time, most school nurses were mature women, who had chosen to work in the school health field because the commitment matched commitments to their young or growing families, and because in most instances it meant they worked school hours, as well as having school holidays. They were inclined to fulfil their role and functions effectively while on the job, but had little or no professional involvement outside. The limited image was compounded by the priorities of dealing with infestations and infections, and the heavy burden of treatments of minor ailments. Few outside the school health field appreciated the positive effects such efforts had, nor were there any moves to enlighten the clientele and general public. It was somehow assumed that others would know what school nurses did and were – by osmosis? Additionally, many school nurses were so involved in dealing with large-scale problems, that they rarely established interpersonal relationships with pupils or teachers, and when youngsters left school they perpetuated their perceived image of the 'nit-nurse'. Image-building was not helped by the fact that within the staff structure, as recognized and negotiated by the then Whitley Council for Nurses and Midwives, the name 'school nurse' did not feature at all, and those authorities who wished to employ experts in school health had to do this by nefarious means. Few, if any, incentives were provided to develop role or image. It seems almost a miracle – or is it another reality based on facts and determination? – that the present situation has changed so dramatically.

Another fact, perhaps minor but nevertheless relevant, is that facilities for practice were (and in some instances still are) minimal, thereby reducing status and recognition of value. Additionally, in most cities and many counties all public health nurses, including health visitors and school nurses, were expected to wear a type of uniform, or at least appear clad in specified styles and colours. The image of the 'Green Ladies' of Glasgow or the 'Blue Ladies' of Lincolnshire has not totally disappeared yet. Because of the priorities of their work, school nurses, whether they wore uniforms or not, protected their street clothing with white, formal overalls and were therefore seen as figures rather than people. Easy-care materials have been a technological asset to nurses wishing to wear 'normal' clothes and be perceived as people, individuals, as well as professionals. All of these factors allowed other professionals to become patronizing; to perceive the school nurse as a useful cog in the wheel of health care, and enabling them to raise barriers to the successful emergence of a fully competent professional practitioner.

SELF-IMAGE

The first step towards being fully valued by others, is to recognize, develop and demonstrate one's own value, i.e. to present an image of self as one would wish others to see it (Berne, 1975). School nurses of the 1980s have the competence and confidence to do this. Each school nurse should see herself as a competent professional practitioner, though recognizing the parameters of and limitations to any independent actions, such as accountability and referral of matters beyond one's competence. The self-image should include acknowledgement of the ability to reach decisions, be involved in decision-making with others, and the capability to make professional judgements, based on data and information. It should also include a realization that each practitioner is a role-model, and that each individual has to be aware of the presentation of self. The latter was described in some detail by Goffman many years ago (1956), but remains as relevant as ever.

School nurses must also overcome their remaining reluctance to present themselves as able professional persons instead of subservient or ancillary staff, or as second-class citizens because either they see their professional role as secondary to their private ones, especially as 'wife' and 'dependent', or because they still feel themselves as such in the dichotomy of their role as a woman. It is not suggested that self-image should develop into a 'holier or better than' others projection, but that it at least does not underestimate intrinsic and extrinic values, and recognizes that it is equal to others who may be more expert at image projection, or who may just be capable of 'shouting louder'.

Image projection

Once the self-image has been successfully established and gives a positive feedback for progress, it becomes important to project this and inculcate it in others. The initial phase is to enable others to recognize the competence inherent in the practice of school nursing. This can be done by 'playing the game' (Berne, 1968), i.e. in the current situation by providing quantitative evidence of success. It is acknowledged that statistics and other data are open to a variety of interpretations, and often such interpretations are made to fit into existing or preconceived patterns. It is therefore a corollary that the quantitative evidence is interpreted by school nurses in the way they perceive its meaning and value, and that their interpretations are publicized, together with or additional to other statements. The second phase is to provide and promulgate qualitative data. This is much more difficult, as such data are often subjective, are based on value judgements and considers base-line data in the light of other factors and evidence. Some qualitative evidence should be based on research, not necessarily the type of research carried out by academicians but, equally validly, action research based on observed and measured practice.

To date, a few school nurses are actively involved in providing the qualitative evidence needed for image projection; others are contributing to full-scale researches and some are considering the application of research evidence to practice. There are also some who are starting to publicize their findings, though unfortunately not yet in sufficient numbers to be overwhelming. It is one area of regret that many school nurses are producing splendid research projects as part of their training courses, but that nearly all of them remain the exclusive property of the individual or the examining institution. Any piece of research, however small or extensive, good or limited, which is part of a qualifying examination has to remain confidential to those concerned until such a time as the course and all its elements are completed. Some Training Institutions require that such pieces are kept confidential until all students, including referred or deferred candidates, have completed examinations and any required additional course work. At the end of such periods the project can be returned to the author, or, as happens more often, is placed in the institution's library. The means of collating and publishing this growing body of work are limited; however, it should be possible to inaugurate an index available to all those interested or to negotiate with specialist central libraries, such as those of the Royal College of Nursing or the Health Visitors Association to stock copies of the projects, and make them available as part of their general services. Whatever the means adopted, the time seems right to utilize this useful body of evidence.

In considering self-image above, several points have been made which also form part of image projection. Additionally, a measure of assertiveness is also required; not aggression or attack on others' professionalism, worth or image, but a positive contribution establishing the school nurse's place in professional life and society in general. Such self-projection should indicate the place in the established pecking order, or hierarchy, which is seen as most appropriate by the person projecting the image. A self-effacing, withdrawn kind of approach is often perceived as not meriting attention or credit; a too forceful approach may be seen as counterproductive. The relationship of self-awareness, including self-image and image projection, was recently described by Bond (1986). In her guide for nurses she also deals with the stresses which may be engendered, and (in Chapter 5) the assertiveness which may be more than useful to establish and project a positive self-image.

SELECTION FOR SCHOOL NURSING

Selection for school nursing is based first on choosing between those people who may apply or are available for the posts, i.e. those who see themselves as potential school nurses. Motivation for applying is usually mixed, as it is for most jobs. It will include the applicant's perceptions of the post; the model or image which has been presented to her before completing any application form, for example, the image gained while on community experience during general nurse training; the prospects envisaged for career advancement or job satisfaction; and, in many instances, a view of self in that role which may or may not be realistic. Chronological age has no direct relevance to which factors predominate, though it may affect the range of motivation and perceptions.

It appears, from scanty existing evidence, that the youngest, most recently qualified nurse, and those who have been in a prior occupation for a very long time, are likely to be those who have the greatest number of preconceived ideas or prejudices, and are likely to find it hardest to adapt to a changed image and role. The latter seems obvious, the first is more surprising until one considers the limited experiences to which most nurses are exposed while undertaking general training in sheltered, hospital settings. It also appears that many newly qualified general nurses have not yet outgrown their adolescent attitudes (white or black, no shades of grey) or that sharp contrasts, which bear so little resemblance to reality, have been reinforced during their initial training.

The applicant may also bring images which were experiences of her own schooldays, or those reported by her children. It seems that those whose experiences were totally negative are unlikely to become applicants; however, it has been noted at some interviews that some people apply with a view that they would wish to improve on the job as perceived in the past, and that they do not wish to expose future generations to their own experiences.

Second, selection is based on the perceptions of the selection panel, or individuals within the selection and decision-making team. The selectors may have specific personal qualities in mind which they see as being essential for the offered job; they certainly will require proof of initial qualification and be interested in prior experience and knowledge. They are likely to explore the attitudes brought by the person and try to assess whether these would in any way adversely affect the functions within the post. They should also be concerned with basic competences, though they may offer posts with the proviso that they are subject to following approved training courses. There have been a number of studies into processes of selection, and the outcomes appear to suggest that the same factors are determined whether the interview is long or short, structured or open-ended or conducted as a solo performance or a group session, provided that the interviewer is skilled at the task. Many selectors predetermine criteria for selection so that they can assess applicants on a reasonably fair scale, and can indicate, if requested to do so, where they see deficiencies or additional attractions.

The other interesting discovery made by researchers into selection procedures is that, whatever the criteria and whatever the job in hand (the researchers looked at diversities as great as the Ford Motor Company and the Civil Service), selectors have a subconscious desire to choose people who may perpetuate their own image, i.e. they are likely to select those who most resemble their own perception of themselves (Goodland, 1984; Open University, Social Science Course).

In most selection situations references from previous employers or other responsible people form part of the procedure, though many references have little real value. It has become established practice to require specific information as part of any reference in an attempt to create relevance, and to structure this information. In many interview situations the gaps left by the application form and in the content of references form the basis of the discussion, as they are likely to form the crux of the decision-making process.

It has been traditional, especially in nursing, for selection interviews to be a one-way process, the selector playing the dominant role. This is another tradition which is changing rapidly and positively. The applicant should select the place of employment and interview prospective employers as well as assessing the offered employment situation. It requires some preparation to face an interview with pertinent questions in hand, and some confidence and courage to request to view the prospective place of employment. Some nurses are still inclined to feel intimidated, and believe that asking questions will count against them. There may be some employers who feel threatened by thoughtful employees, but most will welcome an approach which should demonstrate the ability to initiate action, and which shows sufficient interest to consider the offered post as a permanency and not as a stop-gap. It would also show that the applicant is informed as much as possible about the parameters surrounding the post and should therefore be able to adapt to the given situation.

In summary, the two major elements to selection are the self-image of the applicant and the professional image desired by the employer, with the themes of competence, confidence and ability as supporting evidence, and knowledge, experience and qualification as base-lines.

SELECTION FOR TRAINING

Post-registration education and training is based on many of the criteria used for selection as an employee, with the addition of academic ability or the determination and inherent ability to work at course requirements. During the early years of courses in school nursing, the main criteria for selection was being a postholder and being seconded or financed by the employer. This created a few dilemmas, in that it was difficult and personally destructive to fail or defer a person who had in other ways been judged as competent to carry out the role and functions, and been accepted as a colleague in the various teams. The situation did not arise very frequently, but when it did a variety of escape routes were opened, for example the person was given the opportunity to withdraw from the course, thus avoiding the stigma of failure, but leaving the employer to devise methods and means of enhancing competence. Alternatively, the assessed practice component of the course could be increased until the person was assessed as sufficiently competent. These dilemmas led to the present situation where most training institutions require the prospective student to give an indication of her potential, either by completing an entrance test or by selection through interview.

Many school nurses have fears relating to their abilities in completing an academic course, with the introduction of new subjects, an extension of their present state of knowledge and the need to perform well in whichever scheme of assessment is used. Among the generalized fears are a dread of having to produce written work, often after a gap of quite a few years, and of encountering new methods of teaching and learning such as participative workshops and other experiential modes, when previous experiences have been didactic, i.e. lectures with as little discussion as possible; not least is the fear of being in contact and competition with peers. In general, these fears have proved to be groundless, the challenges of new materials have been welcomed and created demands for more. Assessments have shown no lack of ability but instead a tremendous amount of previously hidden talent. The greatest boon has been the break with professional isolation and the sharing of knowledge and experience with others, even if mild competition stimulated greater effort. The production of written work has had to be circumscribed, as so many course participants produced a quantity and quality of work in excess of demand, and more importantly in excess of the time available for producing and marking it. Some did not find it easy to regress to being a student, though most have found it a welcome break from the stresses of the daily round, and even more a welcome opportunity to stand back from their work and look at it objectively. The outcome has been renewed strengths and for a substantial proportion of people, a whetting of the appetite for more which has led them to other courses and other studies.

Currently, more than 50 per cent of entrants to courses have minimal experience as school nurses; they are selected with a commitment to undertake training, the commitment being on both sides, employer and employed. Course leaders have found it beneficial if the student has some background experience in the community, and some familiarity with the ideas and concepts she is likely to meet on the course. Many courses supply a pre-course reading list, so that stress can be reduced; many prospective students request such information, though few actually manage to do more than scan the proffered material – just proving that school nurses *are* human.

FAMILY IMAGE AND SUPPORT

The ability and capability of most school nurses is no longer in doubt. Selection procedures for employment and training reflect the present – hopefully. The difficulty few expected to face, but many have reported, is that their families reacted in unexpected ways to their enhanced status and proven ability. There are, of course, as many permutations as people, but a few examples can be given. Many husbands are willing to accept that their wife takes on a job, but they resent the job when it leads to professionalism, to commitment and to the confidence which this brings. They also worry if they believe that the professional role will lead to neglect of other roles, and find considerable difficulty in adapting to change, and even more difficulties in changing ingrained attitudes. Such concerns can inhibit the nurse's development, on both personal and professional levels, and lead to her not achieving either her potential or job satisfaction. In complete contrast, some husbands are proud of their spouse's achievement and will provide whole-hearted support, despite any changes this may entail. Nurses with a positive family support system are usually enabled to develop successfully.

Children of many ages have also reacted in many different ways to their mother's image as a professional. The initial reaction is usually surprise that Mum can do more than just look after the family; often the reaction is fairly self-centred in that the mother's professional role is judged by how little it affects her youngsters. In the long-term there is usually pride, and often relief, in that the professional attitude of the mother spills over into the home situation, and leads to diffusion of much tension. Many teenagers have been amazed and thrilled to study together with their mothers, at the same time and often sharing the same table, but each following their own subject matter. The resulting discussions and debates have generally added another dimension to family life, and made it more dynamic and positive. Many school nurses do not have either husband or children, but still have the responsibility of other dependent relatives, most commonly elderly parents. It is often difficult for elderly parents to regard their daughter as anything other than their child, and the professional role is fairly meaningless. However, they usually approve of achievement in whatever terms this presents itself, and are normally aware of the daughter's need to be a wage-earner. Varying on the degree of dependency, this does not always mean that they abate demands. School nurses with dependent relatives, that is, those attempting to combine the role of professional with the role of informal carer, often experience considerable stress; this may inhibit performance either in the work or in the learning situation.

IMAGE OF THE SCHOOL NURSE AS AN AGENT OF AUTHORITY

School nurses are often seen as representing authority. The nature of the authority varies as to whether it is perceived as being inherent in the role of nurse – equated with the authority figure of a ward sister – or as representing the establishment: 'Authority'. In either event this is a perception which includes measures of respect and expectations that the person will act accordingly, be full of wisdom and possess knowledge, which is impossible or unlikely that any one person will actually hold. Some people find such an image gives them a protective shell which they welcome; others find that it can create barriers. It is a normal human reaction to respond to the perception of others; in this instance the responses span a spectrum of total acceptance to great efforts to be seen as an equal. Reality appears to lie somewhere in the centre of the spectrum; a total authority figure is likely to create barriers to effective communications. There are times when the explicit or implicit authority of the role has to be used, e.g. when excluding children from school because of infections or infestations, and there are times when equality or partnership is more productive than any other approach. It is also likely that the position of the person on the spectrum will vary with each situation, through time and in different settings. It can therefore form a dynamic aspect of the role and functions.

Being seen, or seeing oneself, as an authority figure is not the same as being authoritarian; the latter means having an inherently dogmatic, inflexible attitude which is convinced of the 'rightness' of held opinions and actions, and the expectation of the person that their opinion will be acceptable to, and seen by others as the answer to all questions. It usually denies or denigrates the value and opinion of others.

IMAGE OF THE SCHOOL NURSE AS A GOVERNMENT AGENT

Irrespective of the beliefs or political opinions held by individual nurses, all those employed within the health, education or social services can be perceived as being government employees, at local or national levels, or state officials. The contract of employment follows national agreements and guidelines, and the wages come out of the public purse, the Treasury, whether they are actually administered by local government authorities or through the largest government department, the NHS. The framework which governs and regulates nursing is a national one, to which the Secretary of State has to be a signatory, and some of the functions are enshrined in national legislation. Every nurse has therefore the same legal obligations as any law-abiding citizen, and additional ones related to her sphere of work. In the first place this means that anyone who is not registered as such but claims to be a nurse can be prosecuted; second, it means that many nurses may find themselves in a conflict situation in holding, sometimes strongly, opinions which contrast with established policy. Each occasion requires decisions, which are usually personal ones, of whether to accept the existing situation, whether to take legitimate steps to attempt to influence and change it, or whether to opt out. The most important factor is to be aware of the framework within which one operates at any given time, whether it is deliberately or incidentally designed to manipulate people within it, and to what extent and by which means it is itself open to manipulation. There also has to be awareness of changes in the framework and political influences which may affect operant levels. Most nurses see themselves as members of a caring profession, and as being professionally responsible; they forget about being part of the Establishment unless it becomes an irritant. In fact, each nurse employed in the public sector is a government agent, irrespective of which political party leads the government, and is therefore subject to the advantages and disadvantages this entails. School nurses are no different to their colleagues from other branches of nursing, but they may be affected more profoundly as government policies of all sorts affect the client groups in the community more directly and often more immediately than is apparent in institutional settings, such as hospitals, which provide havens for short periods of particular need.

An inherent dilemma in being a government employee or agent is the official expectation that government policies will be promoted, as well as accepted and implemented. There appear to be many situations when policies are accepted because that is a legal requirement, but with a view to effect legitimate change or as a temporary measure. The question of promotion of policies is a more open one. Each person has to decide when or whether they actively participate in helping to advance or promote proposals and ideas, and when they fulfil only their legal obligations and no more.

IMAGE OF THE SCHOOL NURSE AS AN AGENT OF CHANGE

School nurses are involved daily in intervention techniques, whether these consist of health education or health care plans to alleviate an identified condition, preventive measures such as immunization or advice on specific aspects of healthy living. Each one thereby becomes an agent of change in relation to the individuals with whom she deals.

This concept can be applied to whole communities, i.e. the population of whole schools and thereby of a district or geographical area, and can involve decisions based on ethical and moral considerations (Rumbold, 1985). Intervention and change may be desirable, but the degree of influence or persuasion used must be balanced with the freedom of each individual, each person's right to make decisions about themselves, and the boundaries to be acknowledged when affecting others' lives. At times balance also has to be sought in affecting change in individual lifestyles, and attempting to change attitudes or behaviour patterns within groups or communities. Nurses can effect change at many levels; they must do so only with complete awareness of how they are achieving this, the means and methods used, and the wider effects of any change. They must continually concern themselves with the question of when intervention becomes unwarranted interference, and when intervention may be contrary to integral values and beliefs. The latter becomes increasingly complex when working and living in a multicultural society. Teenagers in many schools may react to proposed intervention by aggressive or violent behaviours. School nurses must develop the ability to recognize potential violence and diffuse aggression (Weiner & Crosby, 1985).

IMAGES HELD BY OTHER NURSES AND OTHER PROFESSIONALS

At the beginning of this chapter the image and self-image of school nurses was considered. It is also important to consider how others see school nurses. One striking fact seems to be that everyone perceives other people's roles and functions differently from the way they perceive them and/or themselves. On many occasions this is the crux of miscommunication. Each professional group is aware of the image which it wishes to project, of the changes which have occurred within it through time and development, but each group also has perceptions of others which may be rooted in the past, on good or less good experiences, and on the interface of the group with others.

Few groups are totally aware of the changes occurring in other groups, or the rate of change to which they may be subject. Nursing colleagues may therefore still perceive school nurses as people who have taken temporary jobs to meet family demands and needs, not as fully active and competent members of a specialist and developing group; few nursing colleagues will have more than superficial awareness of the totality of the sphere of school nursing. Other professions may be even more vague.

Teachers are likely to base their perceptions of school nurses on the experiences within their schools, and therefore on the ambassador of the profession with whom they have had most contact. It is pleasing to record that recent reports indicate very positive images among many teachers, but the stage of total acceptance of the desired image has not yet been reached. Education Welfare Officers, Social Workers, workers from voluntary agencies and specialists in many other disciplines all depend on their image of school nurses on those whom they have met, or on the fact that they rarely meet and therefore base their perceptions on their own childhood or the mass media. If the last is of the soap opera kind, for example 'Angels' (shown on TV in the 1980s), it is likely to contain many mythical or fictional elements.

The general public – our clientele – normally has only the image of a bedside nurse, reinforced by novels and other forms of available literature. Only time and continual personal education will assist a wider understanding of preventive, promotional nursing care in the community.

Medical Officers and other medical practitioners also vary in their perceptions. A surprisingly large number only perceive others as they wish to perceive them, i.e. in relationship to themselves as individual practitioners, and they have minimal constructs of others' reality. Some have an image of all nurses being first-year students and conveniently forget that most have developed into competent practitioners without any form of dependence on medical influence. Some are striving to form realistic and positive professional relationships, and welcome a team, i.e. an equalitarian and partnership, approach, and still others work closely with school nurses and fully appreciate their value and share their own image of themselves.

All this demonstrates the variety of perceptions and images which are held by a great variety of people, and that this is an area which must be kept under active review and consciously developed. Many of the facets of school nursing discussed in other chapters of this book contribute to the images projected and held. Perceptions are slow to change, and sometimes suffer periods of reversal. The foundations are now sufficiently secure to provide a basis for building into the future and for any remaining negative images to be overcome.

SUMMARY

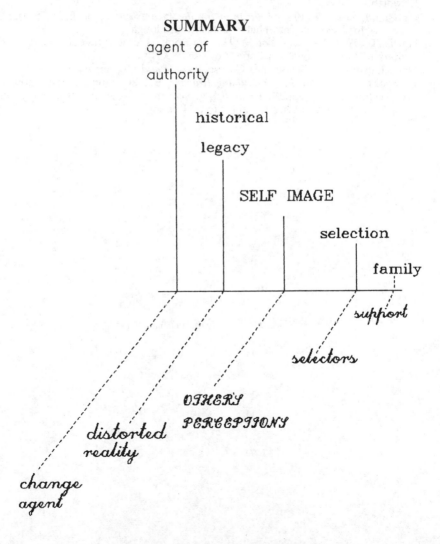

REFERENCES

Berne, E. (1968) *The Games People Play – The Psychology of Human Relationships*, Penguin Books, Harmondsworth.
— (1975) *What Do You Say After You Say 'Hello'? The Psychology of Human Destiny*, Corgi Books, London.
Bond, M. (1986) *Stress and Self-Awareness – A Guide for Nurses*, Heinemann, London.
Goffman, E. (1956) *Presentation of Self in Everyday Life*, Pelican Books, Harmondsworth.
Goodland, S. (ed.) (1984) *Education for the Professions* (especially Chapter 3), Society for Research into Higher Education, Slough.
Harris, T. (1973) *I'm OK – You're OK*, Pan Books, London (first edition 1970, *The Book of Choice*, Jonathan Cape, London).
Open University, Social Science Course, *People and Organizations*.
Rumbold, G. (1985) *Ethics in Nursing Practice*, Ballière Tindall, Eastbourne.
Weiner, R. & Crosby, J. (1985) *Handling Violence and Aggression*, National Council for Voluntary Child Care Organizations, London.

11
HEALTH EDUCATION IN EDUCATIONAL SETTINGS

Health Education is a term which covers a vast range of activities. It provides those who believe in its value with the means towards health-enhancing behaviours, towards improved lifestyles and a strong force in preventing ill-health or deterioration. There are some who see it as a panacea for curing all ills, medical, educational or social, and some who see it as a tool for achieving renown without getting too personally involved. Others see it as a proscriptive medium, which is used solely to discourage them from enjoying life and its few pleasures. The name itself spans two major disciplines and often falls between two worlds, health being unromantic and boring – until no longer available – and education holding some pejorative connotations.

Reality falls somewhere between these different perceptions. It seems certain that health education, if properly and appropriately presented, can give the information and knowledge as well as some life skills to make decisions which improve health and thereby the ability to enjoy life. Health education as part of the school curriculum can assist in preparing young people to become good parents and citizens, as well as physically and mentally able to cope with a range of situations. Health education in the work place can lead to the avoidance of accident and injury. Health education for those already suffering from a diagnosed condition, or for their informal carers, can give them the means to improve their chances of recovery or prevent deterioration. Health education can provide information on new developments, research findings or the causative factors of diseases. At its best, health education can provide each person with the range of available options to make their own decisions about the life they wish to lead in terms of their own and their families' health.

There are quite a few things health education cannot achieve. It cannot cure all social ills nor can it cure established disease or handicap. It cannot, and should not, enforce its message, but allow people to make their own decisions in full knowledge of possible consequences. It cannot conjure up health when other conditions, such as polluted environment, dirty water, overcrowded accommodation, poverty or unemployment, mitigate against it.

Health education can be practised – by those who are qualified professionals and by knowledgeable members of the public – with skill and wisdom. Equally, it can be abused by people to manipulate others or to create a political climate for their own advantage. The dangers of this were discussed by Strehlow (1986) in a paper presented at the First International Conference on Health Education in Nursing, held in Harrogate in 1985.

HEALTH EDUCATION IN NURSING

Health education as an officially recognized entity has undergone many phases. Job descriptions of nurses and others working in the community have contained a teaching element for many years, and their preparatory courses have attempted to give them the base-line for practice. The syllabus for general nurse training, 1977, includes preparation and practice of health and patient education, based on the Nurses Rules (1976). The role of every nurse, at whatever level and in whichever setting, as a health educator is gaining greater recognition, though there continues to be a gap between aims and reality. Several surveys have shown that implementation of the 1977 syllabus is not equal everywhere (Faulkner, 1985; Health Education Council, 1980).

During the 1970s there were attempts to professionalize health education, and health education officers were appointed with a variety of backgrounds and variable preparation, as well as very varied resource and support systems. Health education facilities and their officers currently form part of each district and provide a useful resource for personnel from health, education and social services as well as devising, originating and co-ordinating programmes and materials (Health Education in Schools, 1983). There is greater recognition that no one person is qualified to carry out the whole range of tasks and teaching, and that no one is *the* expert. There are people of many disciplines who hold the Certificate in Health Education, validated by the Health Education Council (HEC) and an increasing number who hold higher educational qualifications up to and including degree level. Most of the degree options are open to those from nursing backgrounds; it is not clear whether any school nurses have availed themselves of this opportunity to date.

Recent publications from the Royal College of General Practitioners and other medical sources (Faculty of Community Medicine, 1986; Royal College of General Practitioners, 1985) urge medical practitioners to take greater cognizance of their health education role, especially the opportunistic one inherent in every consultation. There are some who have taken this message to heart and developed means for health education within their day-to-day practice.

Teachers, as the prime educators, have always carried a responsibility for health education, though this was implicit for most and not part of their subject matter. In most schools some teachers have become the recognized 'experts', either as part of human biology, physical education, home economics or civics, which appears on timetables under many guises. A core of teachers have developed a range of courses and programmes, whose subject matter is specifically related to health and wellbeing. The Department of Education and Science through their in-service education programmes and the Schools Council produced materials and courses to help teachers in this subject area. Since the demise of the Schools Council, materials are being produced by the Health Education Unit at the University of Southampton and the HEC, among others. Much generally available material is concerned with the teaching of health matters, to the extent where it is not easy to discern the wheat from the chaff, nor the most appropriate for any age-group or setting.

Health education should be a part of every nurse's role and function. It is a fact that nurses working in hospital settings may have patient education as their priority, i.e. education on how to cope with specific diseases and their consequences, or how to adapt to and cope with a disability or handicap resulting from disease. They should be able to accept their broader responsibilities of educating patients' families, and of some preventive education to minimize repetition of many conditions and avoid others; they also have the inherent responsibility of providing health education for other professionals and colleagues and acting as role models.

Nurses working in the community have health education as one of their prime functions, though their role may place differential emphasis on its nature and extent. In summary, Occupational Health Nurses are likely to concentrate on education related to the adult working population and make accident prevention one of their priorities, though they may be closely involved with a range of health-oriented campaigns, preventive measures and citizen or family life education. Like others, their recent concerns include alcohol and solvent abuse, violence in society and its effects, and not least avoidance of the spread of infection, including the acquired immune deficiency syndrome (AIDS) and other sexually transmitted diseases.

District Nurses have a very clear function in the education of patients and their relatives. This involves not only teaching about disease and how to cope with its effects, but may also encompass nutrition, lifestyles, exercises for health and recovery, adaptation of the environment, suitable clothing and other material aids to living and concerns itself with preventive education, especially in the field of mental health and the prevention of depressive illness and possible suicide. Many district nurses undertake bereavement counselling and have a strong educative role in this field. More recently, the preventive role of district nurses has become recognized, and there is considerable debate about their involvement in pre-retirement education, preventive health education for the senior adult population who have not yet reached dependent or sickness status, and their contribution to the broader concerns of health education.

Nurses working in family planning and other specialist clinics have specific educative roles, often far beyond the scope of the clinic's subject matter. It is of interest to note that, currently, approximately 50 per cent of family planning clinics are staffed on a sessional or part-time basis by school nurses. It is obvious that the educative role increases when these specialists meet defined groups, such as teenagers or adolescents, and where the subject-specific advice and information has to extend to much broader perspectives.

Health Visitors' educative function should permeate 90 per cent or more of their working life. Their generalist functions provide them with the opportunity to reach groups and individuals of all ages and in a variety of settings, and their professional preparation should enable them to practice health education in a variety of ways. Many health visitors continue to undertake health education in schools, they are certainly involved with parents of schoolchildren, and with teenagers who may have left school or who should be at school but do not attend for a variety of reasons. The subject matter of their educative programmes should and could be as varied as the setting and situation suggests, and may be individualized or follow national or district policies. Health visitor's responsibilities in school settings can best be met by team work with school nurses and others.

HEALTH EDUCATION IN SCHOOL NURSING PRACTICE

School nurses are the health experts in educational settings. They therefore carry a responsibility for health education of the school-aged population, though they share this with teachers, parents, health visitors and others.

Each school nurse has the opportunity for one-to-one health education of pupils in the settings for which she is the named nurse, or which form her area of functional responsibility. Every contact with pupils can provide such opportunity and should be utilized to its full potential. Some of the potential is indicated in Chapter 5 within the discussion on functions. Opportunities also have to be created and plans formulated to incorporate teaching on identified health needs and to cover subjects of topical interest. Decisions have to be made which are based on professional judgement or consultation with others, about whether the identified health education need can best be met by individual approaches or whether teaching plans should be evolved for groups or whole classes, even whole schools.

The least used opportunity, as far as can be perceived by any outside observer, is use of the school environment. The educational setting could and should provide one medium for health education. Notice-boards, common rooms, dining areas and some classrooms could be used effectively as display areas for health-related information. This must be of a nature to attract attention, be topical and relevant to the pupils and, above all, be frequently updated or completely renewed. The nurse using this medium must make herself responsible for the relevance, quality and accuracy of materials displayed. She may obtain them from a range of sources, e.g. the school itself, the mass media, the health education unit of the district, or direct from the HEC or commercial sources.

Such incidental displays could form the basis for more formalized prog-rammes. These could then be formulated on the assumption that each pupil has at least a nodding acquaintance with some health topics. Displays could also form a specific, topic-oriented preparatory guide to organized sessions or a medium for revision of an already covered topic. The siting of the latter displays may be in specified areas, so that it is particularly available to the target group. There is considerable debate about the level and style of display materials. Some people, especially some professionals, consider that all materials should be factual and presented in a straightforward manner. Others recognize the value of attractive presentations, even deliberate errors, while still requiring factual content. Others again feel that presentation should match the age and stage of the potential readers or viewers and may take the form of words or pictures, diagrams or cartoons, drawings with short captions or any other eye-catching method.

It would seem that accuracy is essential, topicality is likely to prove valuable, and presentation can take many formats. Audiences, even very young ones, expect some sophistication, though they may appreciate an oblique approach through cartoons or drawings. Displays do not have to rely on written or printed materials. Young audiences are very used to television and video materials, and may be attracted by modern presentations. Most health authorities have access to some visual aid equipment, and in fact many such systems are currently underused. Most educational settings also have modern equipment available and its use can be negotiated. It is a sad reflection that computer games, which attract such a high proportion of the young audience, do not yet contain 'health games'. This could be a useful medium for the foreseeable future. Several resource packs are now available, e.g. the Open University resource pack 'Health Choices', The Youth Training scheme (YTS) health education resource pack 'Health Matters' and the Health guide written by the OU in association with the HEC and the Scottish Health Education Unit (1980).

Advantages and disadvantages

School nurses as health educators face some particular advantages and some decided disadvantages. The advantages are that they have a captive audience, and that this audience is certainly motivated by self-interest. Therefore any information which relates to children and young people is likely to be acceptable and, at the younger age spectrum, received with great enthusiasm. At the upper age spectrum, interest often is hidden and responses are likely to be more coy. Another factor, which can be turned into an advantage, is that health education which can be applied to self is often a welcome relief from routine academic or examination subjects, or a change from subjects perceived as dull and routine. The older, teenage or adolescent audience is likely to require differing approaches and demonstrate interest in more diffuse subjects, such as interpersonal relationships. The responses, if not coy, are sometimes disconcertingly blunt and require a very open, nonjudgemental attitude on behalf of the teacher or nurse. The disadvantages are that genuine interest has to be stimulated and maintained, that the nurse is not a teaching expert and therefore has to adapt herself to the situation, and that the teaching has to be immediately applicable and relevant. Teaching for future, adult health or family or citizen roles has to be approached gradually and with care.

School nurses can evolve a curriculum of health education to run along-side the normal school timetable. If this is to be most effective it should be negotiated with teachers. The latter, in most instances, can enhance and develop the base-lines provided by the nurse. They are in the position where they are faced with questions throughout the school-day. On many occasions these questions will develop out of previous learning, or as an attempt to clarify previous lessons, including health teaching. In many instances, teachers are involved in clarifying misunderstood or vaguely comprehended health messages. Health education can form an examination syllabus, validated by several organizations, such as the NAMCW, GCE or CSE Boards and school nurses may contribute to syllabus requirements.

The second strand of health education which should form part of the school nurse's plan and may have to precede or parallel the first, is providing health information for teachers. Within any school there will be teachers familiar with health-related matters, but there will also be some whose information is based on questionable sources and who may not recognize the deficit this creates. Various approaches can be used to assist classroom teachers in acquiring appropriate knowledge, without threatening their expertise as teachers in any way. First, they can be party to the planning of the health education programme for their pupils, and thereby acquire the wherewithal to gain up-to-date information and references. Second, they can be invited to participate in any sessions, though it is sometimes difficult for teachers to accept a supporting role in their 'own' classroom. Third, they can be provided with outlines of the content of the lessons or sessions, so that they play their supporting role fully informed. Alternatively, separate health education courses can be offered to teachers, either informally in the staff-room context, or more formally as extracurricular or in-service measures. Last, but not least, teachers can be encouraged to take advantage of the provision made by the Department of Education and Science (DES) which annually provides some short courses on health education.

It would appear that some teachers are unaware of this provision, and that they are equally unaware that the cost of attendance is met by the DES, i.e. not out of school or personal funds. The courses are held at different venues, are usually residential and will attempt to cover various aspects of health education. Some courses are organized jointly with other agencies and other professionals, and are therefore multidisciplinary in nature; some are planned jointly with representatives of trades unions, who have formulated health policies. Normally, schools are circulated with information about courses, though it is not always clear how effective such communications are; details can be obtained from the DES.

SETTINGS

The extent and nature of health education in any one setting will vary, of course, according to the age and ability range of the school population and the health education content of their 'normal' curriculum. It may also depend on current and identified health issues, which may be related to locally determined needs, national campaigns or international concerns. The locally determined needs may include nutrition, hygiene, human development, dental care, interpersonal relationships, availability of resources, use of health care facilities, health care policies affecting members of that community, infectious diseases and their prevention or prevention of their spread, caring for others, accepting responsibilities for one's own health, anatomy and physiology, and a whole range of related topics. It is unsatisfactory for the nurse or teacher and students if teaching occurs as an isolated instant. It is much more positive for all concerned if the health education curriculum forms a thread throughout school years. This enables an introduction to be made to the range of possible topics, and a follow-through at greater depth, as well as essential reinforcement and revision.

NATIONAL CAMPAIGNS

National campaigns may focus on particular concerns, either totally health-related or politically biased. *The* campaign of 1986 concentrated on AIDS and every health care professional is likely to be involved in some way. This particular disease, with all its tragic consequences, appears to be receiving disproportionate attention, and it is likely that there will be 'oversell' and therefore anti-reaction. School nurses must keep themselves informed of the facts, which are changing almost monthly as research is progressing, and be prepared to discuss the real issues as well as the myths surrounding this subject. They should also be conversant with available resources and referral points for advice, counselling and practical help. Both the DES and the DHSS have published guidelines for those working in schools (DES, 1986a, b; DHSS, 1985; Russell, 1986).

Health care professionals should be conscious that any national campaign that focuses on one topic, disease or issue, may affect the resource allocation for the continuing health care needs of the population and that, occasionally, national campaigns are a diversionary tactic to remove attention from other equally vital issues. These may include: increasing poverty and its resulting disease and morbidity; underlying causes of addictions; deleterious effects of increasing prescription charges on women's health, especially mothers of young children; diminishing access to health care facilities through shortages of qualified staff; and, not least, depressive and other illnesses related to unemployment and the lack of employment prospects. The last issue may be a very important one in the school health context. National campaigns are usually designed to inform people on a multi-media basis; there is no proof that such information leads to attitude change, nor that, if attitude change does occur, it will be positive, and not consist of retrenchment or hardening and thereby create further dilemmas. *The* campaign of 1987 is likely to focus on the prevention of heart disease, which continues to be *the* killer and disabler of the 1980s. The UK remains near the top of the international league for incidence of heart diseases, which does not reflect kindly on health care provisions. The centrally determined needs are reduction in smoking, especially among young people (schoolchildren!), healthy eating for all age-groups, more exercise and generally improvements in health-related behaviours. There is no information, as yet, that the 1987 campaign will be made effective by providing alternatives to the antidepressant effect of nicotine, by providing sufficient financial resources for all families to be able to afford a healthy diet (a healthy, well-balanced diet for *each* teenager per week is estimated to cost a minimum of £14, compared with the *total* income of *whole* families on Supplementary Benefit levels of £36 per week (London Food Consortium, 1985), nor that exercise or play facilities will be accessible and affordable to the whole population. The only certainty is that health care workers will be expected to support the campaign.

THE INTERNATIONAL SCENE

International concerns include the prevention of child abuse, and finding the means to identify and help all children at risk. The incidence of reported abuse, including physical, sexual, mental and emotional (also including sexual), and dangerous neglect, has reached epidemic proportions. How much of this is due to greater awareness among public and professionals? How much is due to the victim's willingness to speak out and report? How much is a reflection of the increased incidence of general violence in society? How much is a result of the stresses of modern living? None of this is clear, and may never become clear. The certainty is that each school nurse is likely to encounter instances of abuse or neglect, and will be expected to take appropriate action. Many school nurses will also be involved in providing health education for children that relates to abuse: how to recognize when someone makes sexual overtures; how to counteract potential violence; whom to approach if one wishes to report or discuss suspicious incidents.

School nurses will also be involved in teaching children who have been abused, and be part of the team which attempts to alleviate immediate results and provide the facility to mitigate long-term effects. Health education in the field of personal relationships may deal with affected children, as well as giving young people the tools to form future relationships and recognize family and parental responsibilites. Health education in this arena must also concern itself with the formulation of attitudes – to health, to people and especially to people who may be defenceless and dependent.

School nurses, like their colleagues from other nursing disciplines, are not trained as teachers. They are expected to be familiar with the principles and psychology of learning, will have had some experience of education of patients and families, and will have had teaching practice if they have completed the course in school nursing. They therefore have to acquire additional teaching skills in order to fufil their health education role. It is presumed that each nurse is competent and knowledgeable in the subject matter, health, or takes the responsibility for achieving competence in this, as well as taking action to constantly increase and update her knowledge base. They are not in competition with teachers, but are subject specialists, whose input should enhance the school curriculum. Additional teaching skills may be acquired by attendance at specific courses, for example, refresher courses with teaching components, institutes of further and higher education courses, and/or City and Guilds courses, especially 730 for teachers, or in-service education courses at local health or education service establishments.

Expertise will be acquired only with practice, and enhanced by evaluation (self and peer group) and modification. Not all nurses welcome a formal teaching role, though they accept their one-to-one teaching responsibilities. Many nurses find that they function well in small group, discussion-type situations, but get overwhelmed by large classes. Some also find that they perform better with some age-groups than others. In each instance, personal strengths and deficits will have to be accepted, and means found to work with colleagues so as to provide the full spread of activities. It is perhaps not surprising that some of the most effective teacher-nurses are those who were initially diffident and had to make great efforts to develop their teaching skills and to formulate teaching plans which suited them and their clientele.

The classroom situation presents some factors which affect the teaching role, and which are in direct contrast to those found in the nurse–patient relationship. The most significant is the maintenance of discipline and order. Young people become restive if their interest and attention is not held constantly. Attention span varies with age and ability and distractions to attention are usually welcomed, not ignored. It is not easy to hold a health education session in competition with band practice or a football match! Additionally, older pupils may hide discomfort or embarrassment by 'show-off' behaviours, or be reluctant to be seen to be interested in personal education. This can lead to classroom disturbances, and each teacher-nurse will have to devise means of keeping control, though this does not have to follow the pattern of control set by the form teacher. It appears to be professionally unacceptable for a form teacher to be present as a control mechanism, though he or she may form a useful ally as a full participant in discussions.

CONTENT AND PRACTICE

The theory and practice of health education has been described in several recent publications, and it cannot be repeated in this limited context (Collins, 1983; Coutts and Hardy, 1985; Ewles and Simnett, 1985; Strehlow, 1983; Sutherland, 1979). These references are not exhaustive and may be supplemented by materials related to educational practice and theory, the psychology of teaching and learning, and research reports (Baric, 1972; O'Neill, 1983; Open University, 1971). Any reference list is essentially sketchy, and requires updating as soon as it is produced. Most volumes are available in hardback and paperback form, so that interested practitioners can establish their preferred reference library. Many health authorities have now established resource centres, or created access to existing nursing libraries. The latter appear to continue to be underused by those working in community settings. The range of provision of background, preparatory materials is normally adequate, but accessibility may present a problem, as well as the time required to gain access. Naturally, problems are only there to be overcome!

Materials related to the content of health teaching are as numerous and as variable as the subjects which may be covered. It is impossible to be specific or cover the whole range, but attention is drawn to the useful packs which have been produced (for teachers) on health matters by the Schools Council during 1971 to 1983. Each nurse must take responsibility to vet materials for accuracy and validity, and keep herself informed about subject matters which relate to her course plans as well as her practice. This sounds extremely onerous, but in fact each new document or book adds to the sum total of knowledge, or presents it in a new light. Selective reading, referencing in one's personal system, or cross-referencing in one's filing system, as well as noting for appropriate usage, are required. Details can be studied at a time close to its application. Scanning can indicate validity and value; collegiate effort can enhance and share the honours.

Means and methods

There are a few issues which may affect the utilization of knowledge, or the means and methods used for health education. The first is confidentiality of information. Some materials are circulated to particular professionals before their full publication, or for consultation before completion and final editing. It seems sometimes difficult not to share knowledge gained by these means, but discretion has to be applied and selective use made with due care. Some materials are published with embargoes upon them, which means the content is confidential until a certain date. It is part of professional ethics to retain confidentiality until the given date; the major reasons for embargoes of this kind are to establish equality among recipients, to allow for the vagaries of postal and other communication systems and to ensure that the information is lodged at key, decision-making points and levels before being subjected to public scrutiny and sometimes misinterpretation or misrepresentation.

The second issue is legality relating to information processes. Some research projects and findings are based on identifiable people or sites; publication usually attempts to depersonalize this and not create situations which lead to the embarrassment of individuals or, at its extreme, slander or libel. Some instances, which may form useful teaching tools, are *sub judice* for a period of time, i.e. when the situation or the people involved are subject to legal processes or investigation, or when claims relating to details contained within information are being challenged in civil courts.

There are two instances when aspects of legality have profoundly affected the health education practice of school nurses and others in recent years. The first is the legal action brought by Mrs Gillick to prevent, *inter alia*, methods of family planning being taught in school settings. For a period of approximately two years, health educators were not able to offer unsolicited family planning advice to young people under the age of 16, nor to describe family planning methods or materials without the express, written permission of parents or guardians. This was irrespective of need or demand, and did not recognize the epidemic of teenage pregnancies in some parts of the country. At the end of the period the Court of Appeal decided that Mrs Gillick could not speak for the whole population, but that parents could withdraw their children from particular sessions – in the same way as parents have the right to decide the nature of religious education provided for their offspring. Most health education practitioners, including school nurses, have for many years included family planning as one aspect of interpersonal relationships, neither emphasized nor taken out of context, but presenting the opportunity for young people to be fully informed and act responsibly.

The second instance is still working its way through legal and parliamentary systems. It relates to the publication and use of texts which explain different sexual practices, such as, for example, homosexuality.

One body of opinion insists that pupils should be fully informed, and thereby be enabled to form positive and tolerant attitudes, about all aspects of sexuality which they may encounter in their adult life. In contrast, there is the equally firmly held opinion that pupils should be protected from knowledge which may conflict with established moral codes or traditional views of the world. The aspect of this issue which is being debated in Parliament and at local education authority levels is the use of teaching materials, and who should decide the relevance, appropriateness and accessibility of such materials. Health educators are at present in the dilemma that there appears to be no set standard or rule. They may perceive sexual differences as one aspect of human life which should be discussed openly and fairly, without undue emphasis and within the context of discussions spanning the range of possible interpersonal relationships. Their immediate responsibility concerns the relevance and accuracy of the materials they provide or use. It may seem preferable for young people to discuss the range of differences in the relatively sheltered environment of an educational setting, with unbiased materials and educators, than to obtain information and misinformation from other, usually biased, sources.

Health education content and practice is a dynamic process, and it will undergo change even while these words are being written. School nurses are frontline health educators, and should seek every opportunity to enhance their skills and develop this aspect of their role.

SUMMARY

HEALTH EDUCATION

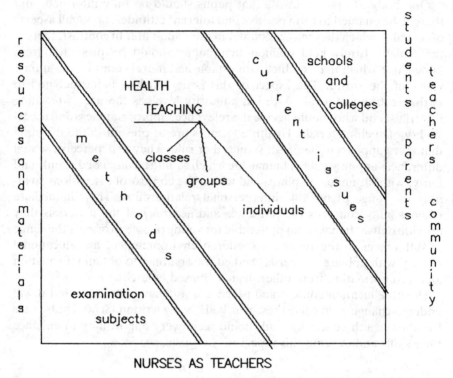

NURSES AS TEACHERS

USEFUL ADDRESSES

Department of Education and Science, Elizabeth House, York Road, London SE1.
Health Education Council, 78 New Oxford Street, London W1.
National Extension College, 18 Brooklands Avenue, Cambridge CB2 2HN.

REFERENCES

Baric, L. (1972) *Behavioural Science in Health and Disease*, Health Education
    Council, London.
Collins, M. (1983) *Communication in Health Care*, C.V. Mosby, St. Louis.
Coutts, L.C. and Hardy, L.K. (1985) *Teaching for Health: The Nurse as Health
    Educator*, Churchill Livingstone, Edinburgh.

DHSS (1985) Circular HC(85)17 *Infection Control Guidelines for the Community Care of AIDS Patients and Other HTLVIII-positive Clients*. DHSS, London.

DHSS (1986) Circular CMO(86)18, HC(86)20 *Guidelines from the Advisory Committee on Dangerous Pathogens*, DHSS, London.

DES (1986a) *Children at School and Problems Related to AIDS*, HMSO, London (in association with the Welsh Office).

DES (1986b) *Administrative Memorandum 2/86*, June, HMSO, London.

Ewles, L. and Simnett, I. (1985) *Promoting Health: A Practical Guide to Health Education*, J. Wiley, Chichester.

Faculty of Community Medicine (1986) *Health for All 2000: Charter for Action*, Faculty of Community Medicine, London.

Faulkner, A. (1985) *A Creative Approach to Nursing*, Ballière Tindall, Eastbourne.

Health Education Council (1980) *Health Education in Nursing: a Survey of Schools of Nursing in England, Wales and Northern Ireland*, HEC, London.

Health Education in Schools (1983) *The Role of the HHS Staff*, North East Thames Region, Health Education Officers' Group, March.

London Food Consortium (1984–1988) *Annual Reports and Monthly Newsletter*, London.

Nurses Rules (1976) HMSO, London.

O'Neill, P. (1983) *Health Crisis 2000*, Heinemann (for WHO), London.

Open University/Longmans (1971) *Personality, Growth and Learning*, OU, Milton Keynes (recently revised).

Open University (in association with HEC and Scottish Health Education Unit) (1980) *The Good Health Guide*, Harper & Row, London.

Royal College of General Practitioners (1985) *Promoting Prevention, Report No. 22* RCGP, London.

Russell, P. (1986) *AIDS in Childhood and Adolescence*, Concern No. 60, National Children's Bureau, London.

Schools Council (1980) *Health Education for 8–10 year olds*, SC, London.

Schools Council (1983/4) *Health Education for 12–16 year olds*, SC, London.

Strehlow, M.S. (1983) *Education for Health*, Harper & Row, London.

—— (1986) Iatrogenesis in Health Education, *Health Visitor Journal*, May.

Sutherland, I. (1979) *Health Education*, Allen & Unwin, London.

12
THE FUTURE OF SCHOOL NURSING

In the present climate of frequent change, considering the future of any individual or any group of professionals is exceedingly difficult in many ways, and to some extent belongs in the realms of astrology. Predictions and opinions are as varied as the people who propound them, often biased towards desired outcomes, and therefore positive or negative according to membership or support of the group under discussion. The following paragraphs will consider the future of school nursing in the light of the current state of the profession, and the existing possibilities and proposals which are in the process of consultation. Outcomes which are perceived as desirable by the author, though they may not follow official guidelines, are indicated in many instances. A few predictions summarize points of relevance and importance made in previous chapters.

INDIVIDUAL PROSPECTS

The major prospects lie in developments within the current role, its extension and progression. In the first instance this means influencing policies so that job satisfaction reflect the desired role, and being very actively involved in formulating job descriptions, their regular review and revision. Each individual nurse has a part to play in this, but the greatest possibility of achieving success will depend on collective bargaining, i.e: influencing by group pressures, irrespective of whether these groups are formed at local levels or whether they represent nationwide opinions and concerns.

Second, school nurses have to develop greater independence from their managers as well as from externally generated influences. Inherent in each case-load is a day-to-day management responsibility. This may be influenced by carefully assessed needs within that load: well-formulated care plans and their concomitant accountability to client and public; availability of resources, including time and ancillary help; maintenance of equipment and its use; health authority policy regarding assessments and procedures; and nationally and locally stated priorities and innovations which are seen by the nurse as essential for continued, competent practice. In the accountability for their own practice, nurses should demonstrate to managers, nurses and non-nurses alike, that they have taken cognizance of all the parameters, and managed their work admirably, thereby becoming relatively independent of personal supervision or interference. External influences include role definitions and perceptions by other professionals, such as medical officers or teachers, accepting and working within others' expectations while defining one's own goals and continuing to work with inadequate resources and materials.

Third, school nurses must gain and demonstrate greater confidence in their role, functions and value. This will assist in the recognition of the role and its functions, and make developments and innovations easier.

Fourth, the concepts of team work, which should lead to an improved service to the school-aged population, should be put into practice. School nurses must play their full part in the teams to which they belong, and take on leadership as well as peripheral roles. As full members of teams they should take part in decision-making processes and in reaching agreements about the most appropriate means and people for providing health care on immediate, short- and long-term bases. They should increase their collegiate relationships with other health care workers, and move towards a partnership approach with clients and public. At present most school nurses are team members with teachers and/or doctors; some are full members of primary health care teams, some are members of nursing teams. However, there are still some who work in isolation. It would appear that the first essential for progress is good working relationships with other nursing colleagues, including health visitors, and extending this to all members of the complete health care team.

Last, and very importantly, it is reiterated that role perceptions, of self, client groups and others, or role image is vital for development. The future must include some active measures to continue the establishment and improve the image of school nursing. Each individual has a contribution to make to this development, both as a practitioner and as a member of a professional group.

CAREER PROSPECTS

Career prospects and their diminution during the 1980s has already been discussed in a previous chapter. The overall aim for the nursing profession has to be to re-establish, albeit in different ways, a career structure and career progression to suit the professionals within it as well as the needs of the 1990s. As part of and contributary to the overall aim, school nursing must define its particular aims in this arena, persuade all its members of the value of such progression, or at least to support colleagues in their endeavours. Currently, those who are active in creating and using opportunities are often hindered by those who should provide most support, even if the latter feel they do not wish to be actively involved.

School nurses must avail themselves of all extant opportunities. In theory there is nothing to block their path to reach top management posts, and any stage in between; in practice there appears to be a conspicuous absence of school nurses above lower management levels. Opportunities must also be created through innovative practices.

There appears to be a politically or economically motivated move towards privatized education. School nurses will have to make their judgements and opinions very clear about the perceived health care needs of pupils and students in any educational system. They may have to decide whether they will remain state employees or enter private competition. In the latter arena they will have to negotiate individualized terms and conditions of service, and their professional organizations or trades unions may or may not have any negotiating rights. It is possible that there will be advantages and disadvantages by working in either system, but any change as profound as this is more than likely to affect roles, career structures and opportunities in many directions.

A move such as the one indicated here could also lead to a split in the school population, more intense than that found in the grammar–secondary school division of previous decades. It is possible that those pupils remaining in the state system will have very apparent, immediate health and social needs, whereas the needs of those in the private sector will only become apparent as unmet when children reach adulthood and make increased demands on health and social services. The provision of school meals and milk, the goods available in school tuck shops and canteens, the general state of nutrition and thereby development of pupils may become crucial issues. It is possible that developmental assessments, including hearing and vision, of pupils in the private sector will become problematic, and that the current state of health of young adults in the UK will deteriorate.

School nurses may be placed in the dilemma of facing not only a professional but also a personal challenge. They may perceive the value of education for all in a state system, but feel that the facilities in the locality where they live are not suitable for their own children, and be drawn towards the private sector, which in turn may require greater financial contribution and make their demands for professional recognition more vociferous! To date none of the protagonists in this debate have clarified how any move will affect those children with special needs, and how any form, however limited, of privatization of education will alter the current move towards integration.

SUPPLEMENTARY CAREERS

There are many bodies and organizations within which school nurses should play an active and contributary part. Some of these activities have to be carried out in addition to normal roles and functions; others can form a temporary or long-term component of the usual sphere of work. Those suggested below are not exclusive, as other opportunities may be equally valuable.

Membership of a health authority

Every triennium health authorities are reconstituted at district and regional levels. Membership is by nomination via the Secretary of State. The exact mechanism of choosing from the list of nominees is not clear to the public, but it should be possible for sufficient school nurses to be nominated for some to be selected on to the authorities. The NHS Reorganization Acts specify the composition of each authority, and the representation of professional as well as consumer groups. Currently, there are very few school nurses serving on health authorities in the category of 'Nurse', nor specifically as school nurses. The range of activities and responsibilities span the whole health district, and include all health service institutions, staff, links with Family Practitioner Committees (FPCs), service and manpower planning, financial allocations and budgeting, and representation on regional and ministerial reviews.

Membership of a Community Health Council (CHC)

Each district has an active Community Health Council, established as part of the NHS Reorganization Acts, and as part of the move towards partnership with the consumer. CHCs determine their priorities depending on the geographical location and the needs within the whole district. They have moved away from the pressure groups which were feared when first established, to become organizations which speak on behalf of health service consumers, which initiate and encourage programmes and activities, and which provide a range of information and advice. There continue to be occasions when members or representative groups of a CHC feel it appropriate to act as a pressure group, usually with good effect. Council members, who are locally nominated and approved by the Secretary of State, may be involved in any or all of the activities, and are in a position to suggest others. One or more members of the CHC serve on the health authority by right, and CHC representatives have the right of inspection of premises, including clinics and surgeries. It is not known whether school nurses are members of any CHC, and if so, whether they are there as school nurses or because they are locally respected as individuals.

Membership of Boards of Governors

Each school and college has a governing body. The representation is supposed to be constituted of the interests within the institution or of concerns which the board of governors is formed to address. The committee is formed from nominated members, though some have to be approved by the Secretary of State as 'suitable'. It is not known how many school nurses actively participate and serve on any of these bodies, as they may be there as parents, consumers or professionals. It is clear that school nurses should know who are the serving members, convening officers and secretaries of their own board of governors, so that they can make their views and concerns known and ensure a hearing at first or second hand. It may imply that those who use the system have to produce written material to present at meetings, but this should safeguard accuracy and avoid misinterpretation. Written evidence does not have to be lengthy; in fact, most busy committee members appreciate short, pertinent, informative documents, which guide them towards decision-making. There also has to be awareness among those who wish to have their voices heard of the timing of meetings and when, or how best, to present their papers.

Membership of other organizations

Membership, especially active membership of professional organizations, is mentioned in Chapter 9. There is a whole range of groups and organizations which require some commitment, but pay large dividends in providing additional resources for the community. Some are specially for women in business or professional life, such as the Association of Business and Professional Women, a national organization with local branches in most cities and many country areas, and the Soroptimist International of Great Britain and Ireland, which is part of a worldwide movement whose first objective is: "To maintain high ethical standards in business, the professions and other aspects of life.' It is interdenominational, with branches throughout the UK which are linked to branches in most other countries. Other associations concentrate on filling gaps in meeting particular needs or leading the way in demonstrating that services should be provided nationally and become generally available, e.g. National Institute for the Blind and the National Association for the Hard of Hearing.

Many of these organizations start life as voluntary bodies, but become government-supported as their worth is proven, for example, the Family Planning Association (FPA). The FPA has many branches throughout the UK which have ceded their original functions to the NHS, and now provide education and training for professionals from many disciplines as well as a large range of educational literature.

The number and names of such groups is limitless; additionally, there are voluntary societies to cover many special needs; some formed for a limited time to achieve particular objectives, others becoming permanent fixtures. The organizations have leaders and officers, some honorary (unpaid), others permanent officials (paid). The officers of any organization form the stabilizing core and provide the links between changing memberships. They should have the expertise to recommend appropriate actions based on experience and previous history of success or lack of such. The officers are usually able to provide the information and its analysis on which decisions should be based. It would be interesting to know how many school nurses lead an active life as members or officers of organizations, and the range of organizations which therefore benefit by their contribution and which in turn might influence the future of school nursing.

MODELS OF CARE

It has become current practice to describe professional practice and the objectives for achievement in terms of models. The names which have become synonymous with models of nursing include Orem (1980), Roper, Tierney and Logan (1985) and Roy (1980). All or any of these can provide a useful framework for practice, as long as it is remembered that they are frameworks and tools, not end-products. To date there appears to be no model of school nursing care and formulation of this could provide one framework for future school nursing practice. It is equally possible that school nurses may wish to study existing models and use the most suitable elements, or decide to reject the current vogue for the use of models as so much 'jargon'. Either of the latter courses of action should be based on a detailed study of the available materials, and a strong argument to those who are convinced that 'models' are the wherewithal to improved care, services and development.

THE NURSING PROCESS

It is not clear whether the nursing process is part of the recent past, the present or the future, though it is clear that the nursing process is something which has currency in debate, and which supposedly is applied in practice by many nurses and incorporated in some health authority policy. The nursing process is a logical, stepwise approach to the provision of care, designed to ensure that all of the patients' or clients' needs are covered and no omissions occur. It involves recording information in an agreed manner, so that all those involved in the care, including the client or patient, can clearly understand the background, current state, influencing factors and the decisions about the actual care, such as what, how, when and who. Any workable process will also include an evaluation or review and reformulation of plans. In the same way as a model, the nursing process is a tool, and it appears to be as effective as the practitioner implementing it. There are instances where the recording element of the process approach has become paramount and has distorted the total picture.

School nurses have not stated publicly whether they consider the nursing process applicable to their field of work, though some have served on working groups within their employing districts and others have struggled with the process approach adopted by their authority. It seems obvious that a process approach can assist in planning and executing effective care, and in clarifying a complex situation. It is not as obvious that the nursing process can be transposed wholesale to a community setting, a school. In the very foreseeable future school nurses will have to decide whether they accept an imposed curative nursing process approach, whether they develop an approach of total relevance to school settings, or whether they accept the use of a process adapted from nursing, engineering or science, but regard it as one method and one tool of their trade. The most nearly definitive text, and one of the few British ones, is the publication by McFarlane and Castledine (1982).

COMMUNITY NURSING REVIEW

The year 1986 has seen renewed activity in policy-making circles to define all aspects of community nursing, to set some objectives and to suggest ways of practice and training for the future. All four UK countries had reviews of community nursing in progress; all four had varying terms of reference, various timescales to complete the task and variable nursing representation.

The English review committee was noteworthy for the fact that it had only one nurse member, and had to co-opt expertise; that it was given six months to undertake a mammoth job; that it concentrated on some aspects of community care and omitted others (in line with the terms of reference) and that it was extremely vigorous in presenting the report to many groups throughout the country. The Report of the Cumberlege Committee was published in May 1986, and the consultation period was due to end in December 1986, though written evidence had to reach the DHSS by the beginning of that month. During 1987 it will become known which parts of the report and its recommendations are to become acceptable to the policy-makers, and will therefore form part of all our futures. The Welsh, Northern Ireland and Scottish reports should also be available during 1987.

The English report has become known as 'Cumberlege', the name of the chairperson of the committee. If the recommendations are interpreted in school nursing terms, and at this stage there are a number of interpretations, it would appear to indicate the following for the future:

1. School nurses would become members of the neighbourhood nursing team, though much work would have to be done to define the neighbourhood. Nowhere within the report is there consideration of how the concept of neighbourhood nursing could be applied to nurses working in comprehensive schools or aligned to the special education and private sector. The report sees the neighbourhood nursing team as complementary to the primary health care team, which is still considered as an ideal state for health care delivery. Nurses of the future will have to work out the communication networks needed.

2. The report does not commit itself to specialist functions, but sees some of the current functions of those working in the community becoming less clearly defined, some might say blurred at the edges, and decisions about the provision of care made on an availability basis. In practice this could mean that school nurses would be involved in the care of sick children – always assuming that they remain child health care specialists. It could

also mean that working hours will have to be renegotiated, to cover the 24
hours of need of a sick child.

3. School nursing was one of the community health care settings which were
   peripheral to the report, and in the little time and opportunity available to
   the committee they could only base their recommendations on inspired
   guesswork. Occupational health nursing, which has so much in common
   with some aspects of school nursing, was not considered at all. These two
   groups of nurses are concerned with health care provision for approximately 65 per cent of the total population.

4. The report's most useful elements are statements about the current state
   of affairs, and some consumer perspectives of preferred means of health
   care, even though there is little appreciation of anticipatory or pro-active,
   preventive health care which is not related directly to age or medically
   defined need. The future of school nursing may be closely tied to more
   widespread understanding of prevention and concepts of health, not
   disease.

5. The proposals relating to the education or professional preparation of
   community nurses made within the report are somewhat vague – the
   absence on the committee of someone with a real understanding of nurse
   education at post-registration levels could be significant. In summary, one
   interpretation of the proposals could be that all nurses working in the
   community should be Registered Nurses (RGN's), that post-registration
   education and qualification would consist of one academic year (i.e. eight
   months) common core with health visitors, district nurses and, at a later
   date, community psychiatric nurses, community mental handicap nurses
   and community midwives. This would be followed by one year of planned
   and supervised practice, including a specialist module. Within the proposals there is no clarity about financial implications for a two-year training
   period for all, no indication of the registration or recording position of
   those who qualify by these routes, or whether such new qualification
   should be mandatory for practice, though there appears to be an implication that completion of training should be a prerequisite for practice. The
   report does not give any indication of the proposed content of the
   academic or practice components; in fact, if this recommendation becomes
   accepted *all* the work related to education and training of the professionals in the community health care services will have to commence,
   leading to further inevitable uncertainties.

6. The Cumberlege committee has urged that implementation of the report's recommendations should begin in 1988/89 and that it should be
   operationalized by 1991. In view of the above comments and the other
   reports and recommendations to be considered in parallel, this seems an

unlikely if not impossible timescale. Some employing health authorities have greeted the report with enthusiasm, some are considering how it could be applied to their settings, and others are regarding it with considerable caution. Even those authorities who are enthusiastic about implementing recommendations within the report are concerned about financial implications, the conditions of service which would have to be re-negotiated, and the grading and salary which may be commensurate with the new type of community nurse (not dissimilar to those working in the 1920s and 1930s). There are some authorities who would prefer to strengthen existing primary health care and other caring teams, rather than move towards new, unknown and unproven entities which are reminiscent of those which were discontinued 20 to 30 years ago because they were ineffective.

7. According to the Cumberlege committee, the intervening period, i.e. the present until the implementation date, should be used to provide updating programmes for existing staff. No firm proposals are made about the nature of such programmes, nor is there any evidence to date that employing authorities have taken notice of this particular recommendation.

8. The recommendations within the report appear to have a range of advantages and disadvantages, and hopefully any implementation will take both into account. The advantages include: parity among nurses working in the community and thereby equal opportunities for career development (if any); less friction between professional groups; more understanding of each other's roles and functions; and knowledge of each other's contribution to the caring process. The extension of education and training facilities will be a welcome proposal for many. The disadvantages include: implementation during a time of economic constraint, when monetary considerations may override any professional concerns and not pay due attention to client and community needs; implementation based on incomplete understanding of health promotion and prevention or the roles and their development of professional carers; conflict with existing and well-functioning teams; diffusion of roles and functions; and dilemmas in meeting crises, as well as curative and preventive needs. The neighbourhood teams as proposed in the report, omit many who currently make a superb contribution in meeting needs and are not clear about relationships with specialist inputs. The proposals are hailed by some as new and evolutionary – possibly revolutionary – however, one could be forgiven for perceiving a re-emergence of Victorian or even Dickensian values, and some concern that, if carelessly implemented, they could prove retrogressive.

PRIMARY HEALTH CARE – A GOVERNMENT GREEN PAPER

At the same time as the Cumberlege report, the government published its intent about the future of primary health care (Government Green Paper Primary Health Care, 1986). The most noteworthy elements of this publication are:

1. Consideration is given to primary medical care; health care is conspicuous by its omission.
2. Where preventive measures are mentioned, these relate to opportunistic advice attached to consultations about ill-health, or to the alleviation and occasional irradication of known diseases. Anticipatory guidance and pro-active primary prevention are largely ignored or misunderstood.
3. Some of the most crucial issues, such as the employment and the role of practice nurses, were stated not to be part of the consultation processes, but subject to ministerial decision only.
4. Parts of the document were addressed to incentives – there was no indication that there would be disincentives for those who did not meet stated objectives, nor that incentives would apply equally to all members of the team.
5. Parts of the document dealt with dental, pharmaceutical and ophthalmic services – the most obvious omission is any form of consumer protection for those services which function independently of national norms or controls.
6. Primary health care nursing was given scant attention; the publication of the Cumberlege report was mentioned and seen as supplementary (or subsidiary) to this document.

The period of consultation is now at its end, and there has been a statement of intent by government representatives to publish a White Paper during 1987. Presumably, this will then become part of the legal framework for practice; at this stage it is not clear what its impact or implications will be.

The most positive proposal within the document is official approval for multidisciplinary post-qualification training and education. Since the late 1960s there have been attempts and many local and national efforts to stimulate interprofessional education for practice, with some successes and some less successful ventures. This appears to be the first occasion where the value of joint learning for those who work together and with similar objectives, i.e. health in the community, has received formal recognition.

The impact of the document on school nursing is likely to be peripheral, unless it is greatly changed as a result of the present consultation and during its passage through the legislative machinery. The main effect is likely to be felt if already scarce resources are further redirected into medical instead of health care.

PROJECT 2000

One month after these documents were published for consultation, the United Kingdom Central Council (UKCC) for Nursing, Midwifery and Health Visiting brought out its project to enable nursing education and practice to meet the twenty-first century with competence and confidence (UKCC, 1986a). The document was the best presented of the three major consultation documents, demonstrating clearly and lucidly the reasons for proposed changes, their possible short- and long-term effects, and giving some indication of what might happen if less radical changes occurred. There were major omissions, such as: details of the content of proposed educational programmes, which were considered to be the responsibility of the four National Boards for Nursing, Midwifery and Health Visiting once the broad principles had been agreed; and the cost and financing of the proposal and the details about phasing and alterations of possible options. The matter of finance, in all its various guises, was placed for detailed consideration with a firm of accountants, which is due to report at the time of writing. A project paper (8 or 9) will be issued in 1987 detailing the consultants findings.

The period of consultation was relatively short, all comments were due to be received by September 1986, as position papers had been circulated during the period preceding publication of the final document, and the profession had been kept reasonably well informed of progress and likely proposals. The project, amended as a result of consultation, and supported (or otherwise) by the detailed financial statements, was due to be presented to the Ministers of Health for all UK countries at the end of 1986. The government's responsibility is to respond and indicate the measure of their official support. The timescale for such a response is somewhat uncertain. Response is expected by July 1987, but it is possible that it may be affected or delayed by the general election.

Project paper 7 has been published recently (UKCC, 1986b) indicating the response received by the UKCC from all branches of nursing. It would appear that the principles within the proposals are welcomed and supported in large measure, but that there are a range of concerns relating to details and implementation. There is one certainty, namely, that change is necessary to meet future needs. It will be uncertain how this change will be effected until all the consultations are completed.

Project 2000 proposes radical changes in basic nurse training and education, based on concepts of health and providing orientation for continuous care throughout the health – ill-health continuum, with much greater insight for all into community-based care. This in turn must have an effect on most post-registration programmes and qualifications, as the person reaching post-qualification level will have a different knowledge base and, hopefully, very different attitudes than many of those emerging from basic training at present. At post-registration level, a module, possibly of two years' duration and containing all aspects of health promotion, is proposed. During basic and post-basic courses there will be common and specific elements, and each will be a mixture of theory and practice, the latter with due guidance and supervision. At the end of the period the practitioner may emerge as a Registered Nurse (School Health) or a Registered Nurse (Health Visiting) or a Registered Nurse (District Nursing), or any similar combination. The post-registration courses are perceived as being at advanced level, with academic credibility, giving those who wish to take advantage of it access to continuing and higher educational studies, including at degree level.

Once it is known how the proposals will be implemented, and when dates are set, there will have to be a massive programme of continuing education for existing staff. As with all major changes, there will be a period where various schemes will have to operate in parallel. For example, there will have to continue to be a post-registration education facility for those who are currently registered nurses or who are currently in training. It will take until the year 2000 to have all schemes completely on line.

The implications for school nursing are therefore likely to be long-term ones; the possibilities are exciting, and it could be one way of achieving complete recognition of value and extent of role. In the less distant future, school nurses are likely to become more involved with trainees at all stages of their preparation. They may have to provide input and experience for those learning about children, and for their development and needs during their basic nurse education. Every trained nurse's educative and supervisory role, including an assessment of competence, is likely to be extended and formally be required as part of normal function. School nurses will be no exception, and may wish to consider this as one step towards a very positive future.

SUMMARY

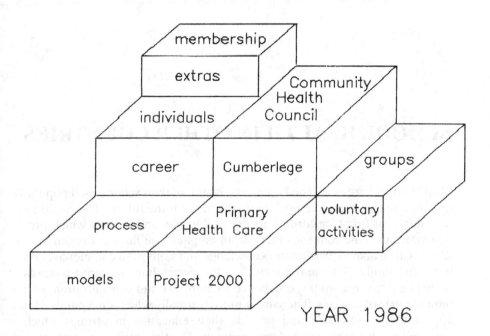

YEAR 2086

membership

extras

individuals

Community Health Council

career | Cumberlege

groups

process | Primary Health Care | voluntary activities

models | Project 2000

YEAR 1986

REFERENCES

Government Green Paper (1986) *Primary Health Care – An Agenda for Discussion*, HMSO, London.

McFarlane, J. and Castledine, G. (1982) *A Guide to the Practice of Nursing Using the Nursing Process*, C.V. Mosby, London.

Orem, D. (1980) *Concepts of Practice*, McGraw-Hill, Maidenhead.

Report of the Cumberlege Committee (1986) *Neighbourhood Nursing – A Focus for Care*, HMSO, London.

Roper, N., Tierney, A. and Logan, W. (1983) *Using a Model for Nursing*, Churchill Livingstone, Edinburgh. Modified in Roper *et al.* (1985) *Elements of Nursing*, Churchill Livingstone.

Roy, C. (1980) *Conceptual Models for Nursing Practice*, Appleton-Century-Crofts, London.

UKCC (1986a) *Project 2000*, UKCC, London, May.

— (1986b) *Project Paper 7 – Results of the UKCC Consultation*, UKCC, London, November.

13
SCHOOL HEALTH IN OTHER COUNTRIES

Most countries are concerned about the health of their school-aged population, and regard it as an important investment for the future. The concerns take different forms, according to the philosophy and politics which predominate. In some countries there is an emphasis on having a population which will be able to provide the knowledge and skills for a commercial and industrial future. This may mean that the curriculum is geared towards discipline in the classroom, obedience to authority and concentration on a limited range of subjects. The same countries usually select some pupils who appear to be most able and provide their education in settings which concentrate on a range of academic subjects. Most countries recognize that learning skills are improved if the physical and mental state of the pupils is such that they can concentrate in comfort and are free from disease. Many of the countries with well-formulated national curricula include physical education as a compulsory subject on their timetables, and subsume health education under this heading.

Physical education, exercises and fitness are seen as being extremely valuable, and there is concerted action to eliminate any reason for non-achievement. Some countries have groups whose beliefs incorporate fitness as a paramount goal; they do not usually see fitness in terms of 'sport', but as a matter for serious attention. The person who provides the regimen for achieving fitness may be a nurse, doctor, teacher or specialist, but responsibility is vested in the head-teacher to ensure that everybody participates. The countries that place most value on fitness of this kind, and will single out for honour those who prove themselves to be most fit, are mainly in the Eastern Bloc and Asia.

The achievement of physical fitness may include recognizable sports, as long as these are not regarded as leisure activities, as well as ballet or acrobatics, which would be considered art forms in other settings. Subsumed within the acquisition of fitness is a recognition that adequate diet, freedom from infection and injury, adequate sleep and rest and avoidance of excesses or substance abuse are essentials. In some instances total control over the life and education of the young person is assumed by the school or other delegated person, with parents playing a very secondary role. The question of diet has a range of connotations, from additional rations of body-building foods to avoidance of meats or vegetarianism, according to prevailing fashion and belief. Because the system relies on 'specialist' concentration to achieve fitness, the role of the nurse becomes secondary unless she is also the recognized specialist, which is quite possible and sometimes the case.

FRANCE

Other countries also concentrate on fitness, but with different emphasis and in different ways. French schools rarely have sports facilities within their grounds or premises, and so children have to travel to participate. The school nurse, sometimes in consultation with the school medical officer, allocates a fitness rating after the school entry examination, and this indicates to teachers and others the amount of exercise or sport which the pupil may follow. The school nurse is the person responsible for amending the rating; for example, a child with a broken limb may be rated zero for a time and, according to the nurse's decision, re-acquire normal ratings as soon as the plaster or bandage is removed, or more gradually. Some teenage girls attempt to obtain reduced ratings in order to avoid sports or fitness activities during menstrual periods. It is the nurse's decision, though she may consult the medical officer or parent about whether there is sufficient cause for a reduction of physical activity, or whether it may enhance coping with stressful times. Many nurses use this opportunity for pertinent, personal health education.

Most European countries, certainly all countries which are partners in the EEC, have official school health commitments. There is great variability in the way they are carried out. France appears to be one of the most advanced countries in this field; school health was declared a national priority some ten years ago. All public services are directed from central government departments, and the departments of education and health in France formulated job specifications for school nurses which are used throughout the country. These oblige the nurse to spend 23 hours a week on health education and health promotion activities in school settings, and the remaining 20 hours on developmental screening and other features of health care. Each nurse has a well-equipped base in school and a defined responsibility for a population not exceeding 3,000 pupils. This could mean one comprehensive school and two middle schools, or several junior schools, or any combination of these. It certainly means that the nurse is well-known in each of her schools, and very much a member of the school team (Strehlow, 1986a). The school system in France is relatively formal. Many buildings are locked during the day and admission is by a member of staff, so that there is complete awareness regarding the whereabouts of any one person, including the school nurse. French school nurses carry complete responsibility and accountability for assessment procedures. The results of these procedures are recorded on the *Carnet*, a developmental and medical record issued to parents for each child shortly after birth. The *Carnet* will show the state of immunization, any accident, illness or injury, and the milestones of development up to and including school-leaving age. At the latter stage, crucial measurements and recordings are made of hearing and sight, and in some instances colour vision. Many prospective employers will consider this record before offering apprenticeships or other posts. The nurse is also responsible for ensuring that any referral is acted upon, and she can demand a written response about actions taken, treatments provided or the reasons why referral resulted in no action being taken. In practice this can mean a communication network spanning many general medical practitioners, as well as a range of specialists and other agencies.

French school nurses who are employed by the Department of Education are usually based in one large school. They assist the Health Department employed nurse in her health education and assessment activities, and provide an onsite treatment service. Treatments can include first aid, dealing with injuries received on the sports field, physiotherapy following such injuries, and occasionally nursing childhood illness, i.e. staffing a sick bay.

Having to spend 50 per cent of working hours in providing health education has resulted in a variety of imaginative interpretations additional to the programmes agreed at district or national levels. Puppet theatres, larger-than-life models, student groups teaching other students, health clubs and film shows are just some of the repertoire. In many instances teachers are involved by the nurse to continue the debate started during health education sessions. A range of materials and handouts are provided from central sources so that health messages can be reinforced.

School nurses in France carry some responsibility for the health care of teachers, and have a definite responsibility for advising about the state of cafeterias and other publicly used areas. They report directly to the head-

Table 13.1 The school nurse: an international comparison

	France	West Germany	UK
Minimum qualification	Registered general nurse and 5 years experience	Registered general or children's nurse	RGN or RSCN
Specialized training and education	May take correspondence course prior to appointment. In-service education started but patchy	9 months' planned supervised practical experience followed by 3 months' course at one of two colleges	3 months' course approved by ENB, leading to recorded qualification
Employer	Health or education department of central government. Appointment by competitive entrance examination	Local authority public health department	District health authority (DHA)
Accountable to	Some districts–nurse manager. Other districts moving from medical officer to nurse management	Doctor, either public health or paediatrician	Nurse manager
Job description	Centrally issued, very detailed, almost prescriptive. Includes 50 per cent of time to be spent on health education	Dependent on immediate supervisor and self-initiated action	Variable
Status	High	Low	Medium
Hours of working per week (full time)	43	40	37.5
Salary level	Senior staff nurse/ ward sister low scale	Staff nurse medium scale	Senior staff nurse or sister medium scale (separate grading)
Conditions of service	Centrally imposed, locally applied	Local, variable. Generally questionable	Negotiated

Table 13.1   *contd.*

	France	West Germany	UK
Working conditions, resources	Very good to excellent	Technically biased, variable	Variable and improving
Career prospects	Minimal if employed by health department	Zero	Increasing possibilities
Job satisfaction	Generally high	Medium, variable	Variable
Major dissatisfaction	Professional isolation	Low status	Adverse working conditions
Professional organization/ trades union membership	Not active	May belong to Nurses Federation, but few do	Increasingly active

tcacher as the frontline manager, but are professionally accountable to senior nurses (school health), with the exception of some country areas where they are accountable to a medical officer (Table 13.1).

GERMANY

School nursing in Germany is officially part of Federal policy, but the provision of services has been delegated to *Lander* (state) or city levels. Many cities are evolving systems of health promotion in schools; other cities find it difficult to allocate resources for any function which is not specified as a legal requirement. All health care in Germany is insurance-based; some 1,200 insurance companies are licenced to underwrite such care. Generally, the companies pay on item-of-service bases, and this does not include promotion of health or prevention of ill-health. It is relatively easy to obtain splendid technical equipment, including the latest in hearing and vision testing equipment, but difficult to get funding for staff salaries if these staff are not involved in active treatments. Additionally, many cities have a plethora of doctors, who in essence carry out nursing tasks, so that the employment of nurses outside the hospital system is not very widespread, nor is it very attractive in terms of career or salary prospects.

Cologne and Hamburg are two cities where school nursing is flourishing. Teams have developed to provide a range of services, including advisory sessions to parents and some large-scale health education programmes.

Caring for children with special needs appears to be a strength in these places. It is perhaps not surprising that school nursing is still comparatively rare in a country like Germany, when one considers that until a very few years ago there was no community nursing service at all, except the emergency and acute service provided by members of religious orders. The first secular course for district nurses was operational in 1981. Two centres, one in the south of the country, one in the north, were established in the 1970s to provide a three-month module following nine months of assessed and supervised practice for school nurses. The courses were medically oriented, though there were inputs on sociology and social psychology. The numbers attending courses were small, and during 1981 there was doubt that the centres would continue to exist; their future is still threatened.

Germany does have a central health education unit which is very active in publishing material for use in schools or with children of school age outside formal school settings. The materials are very detailed, and include all that a person would need to be informed about particular health topics. However, there is a distinct problem. The school curriculum in Germany is planned more than one year in advance, detailing the use of each hour, and it is heavily biased in favour of academic or technical subjects. To include health education in the curriculum, one would have to submit plans for sessions at least 18 months in advance, and be committed to a schedule which allows little deviation.

Those working in the public health field have identified a range of health needs which they feel should be addressed during school years, including hearing deficits, posture modification, nutritional states and a range of behavioural difficulties. Among the last, there appears to be some evidence that attention span among children is decreasing, and that there may be some form of cerebral irritation due to constant exposure to excessive noise levels. This has been noticed in some of the big cities, especially among children who live in high-rise flats, near major roads and are exposed to aircraft noise, not to mention the effects of music, transistors or television.

SCANDINAVIA

Scandinavian countries have well-developed public health services, including school health. The most reported ones are those in Finland, where the young population receives attention from nurses from birth to school-leaving age in a structured and constructive form. The services are organized according to the geographical terrain. In mountainous country areas nurses will carry a curative and preventive responsibility for a small population; in cities the patterns are similar to those found in the United Kingdom. Denmark has some very innovative and exciting schemes, involving school-children in their own health assessment, and was the first country to make children partners in formulating health care plans and taking responsibility for part of their own health care provision.

UNITED STATES

The most vocal group of school nurses originates from the United States of America. School nurses there act more like nurse practitioners, and have a defined role as child protection agents. The reality of being able to fulfil role and functions varies in each of the states, there being in excess of 50 job specifications. Some states have well-defined and active policies relating to school nursing, encouraging health education and innovative inputs in all aspects of the role, which is very similar to that of British school nurses. The child protection role has been strengthened throughout the States, due to the concern with and increase of child abuse in all its forms. School nurses are legally responsible for recording and reporting suspected cases of child abuse, sexual abuse or incest. They take an extremely active part in therapeutic measures designed to help victims, in addition to an obligation to be an expert witness in cases of legal prosecution or care proceedings. Some nurses have expressed concern that their numbers are insufficient to undertake both their legal duties, which they have accepted willingly, and their pro-active, promotion and prevention roles (Kort, 1984). The school nurse is a public employee, which in some states creates tension with the private, insurance-based sector, which predominates in health care facilities. Nurses' status, however, is high: they are regarded as responsible professionals. In some states there is strong resistance to any form of public health, it being seen as unwarranted interference with personal liberties. School nurses therefore may encounter attitudes among their client groups which mitigate against effective practice (Slack, 1980).

SOUTH AMERICA

The Americas, excluding the United States, and many islands and smaller countries which are close to the South American continent, have a confused and confusing school health picture. Some countries, such as Brazil, run a vast network of distance-learning projects. Many young people have no access to school buildings, many more attend irregularly, and some still do not have any formal educational opportunity. It is therefore difficult to determine health input in any of these situations. Health care facilities in many of these countries are as scarce as educational facilities, and usually private and costly. At government levels there is a desire, and some policies, to ameliorate the situation, and certainly health education forms part of the distance-learning school curriculum. Mexico, for example, has some splendid cartoon-style magazines which are entirely free and geared to spreading health messages. Many of the Southern American countries have a few very large conurbations, with all the concomitant problems, and large areas of scarcely populated and often inaccessible countryside. The extremes between rich and poor, ownership of vast estates and excrutiating poverty, and the health that wealth can buy (such as adequate nutrition), compared with the range of poverty-related diseases continue to be apparent. In many instances there has been improved overall provision in the past decade, but the problems are so immense that so far the impact has been small.

Those who function definably as health care workers among the school-aged populations are usually members of religious or other charitable and voluntary groups; often their efforts are confined by their means and ability to move freely among the population. There have been many and prolonged wars, both international and civil, affecting some of the school populations, with resulting traumas, including absence and loss of parents.

In many countries young children become the breadwinners of the family. International agencies have expressed concern about the nature and means by which children earn the money to support their siblings, and often parents and elderly relatives. Begging is one obvious occupation; others include prostitution, both boys and girls, from the age of six or seven years and up; becoming involved in pornographic schemes; and generally being exploited. Recent evidence suggests that child employment internationally is reaching staggering proportions, beyond even the most horrendous reports of earlier years in Europe. Therefore, school health, and school nursing, in these countries is a stated goal, but its achievement is part of the future.

AFRICA

The picture in the developing countries of the African continent is very different and variable. It seems that some countries have made great strides in easing the health concerns related to their school-aged populations. Until three years ago, progress was relatively rapid in most aspects of health care; the recent past has brought severe drought, and all the hazards related to disaster, such as undernutrition and mobility as a refugee. Throughout

Africa there are schools – some provided by the states, some by organizations and societies and a few by private means. All schools concentrate on enabling children to reach their potential as far as possible, and include health teaching in their curriculum. The nature of the teaching has to be very different to that in Western countries, as it often relates to using the environment to its best advantage, to overcoming superstitions and very ancient customs, and occasionally to overcoming apathy.

Most African countries have a great pride in their peoples, and will endeavour to provide the best possible facilities for their next generation. The provision of school health care is variable according to the State and its economic and political development. In most instances the actual care is provided by specially trained local people, who understand the language and customs of the people. These trained lay workers are accountable to a central organization, either nursing or medical, and will both bring and take ideas for further development. The most noteworthy achievement, in a relatively short time, is the irradication of many infectious diseases, including malaria. Measles, which is a nuisance to the children of Europe, used to be a killer when combined with the climate of Africa; the incidence was reported to be reduced by 75 per cent – before the drought.

Poliomyelitis crippled many children and killed some each year, until recent years. Since 1980 there have been only minor instances, with few resulting permanent handicaps. The greatest cause for concern is nutritional disorders of all kinds, excepting obesity, and although progress is fair in difficult circumstances, there is still a long way to go. Many countries of Africa would like to have a school health service similar, though different, to that in Britain, but it has to remain an aim for the future until immediate crises are overcome.

Since its inception in the 1940s, WHO has been concerned with the health of schoolchildren, and through membership of related organizations such as UNICEF and the Children's Centre in Paris, has promulgated health care and health education. Many successes have been possible through support by these organizations; many concerns have been highlighted by them and therefore received public attention and it is certain that their work will continue and stimulate international efforts (WHO Technical Report Series, 1975–85).

SUMMARY

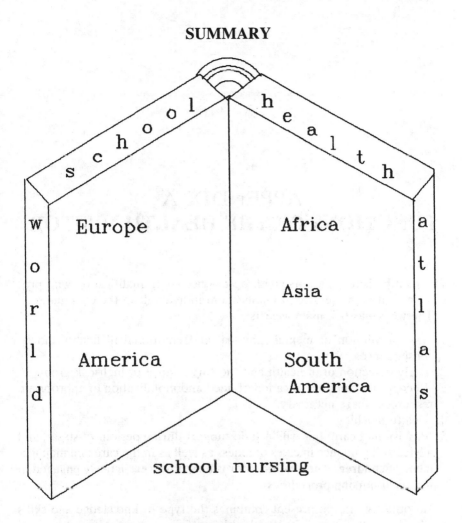

REFERENCES

Kort, M. (1984) The delivery of primary health care in American public schools 1890–1980, *Journal of School Health*, December, *54*, pp. 453–456.

Slack, P. (1980) School nursing in the USA, *Nursing Times*, February and March.

Strehlow, M.S. (1986a) School health in France, *Health at School*, April, *1* (7), pp. 229–230.

— (1986b) School nursing the French way, *The British Journal for Nurses in Child Health*, November, *1* (9).

WHO (1975–85) *Technical Report Series*, WHO, Geneva.

APPENDIX A
FUNCTIONS OF THE HEALTH VISITOR

The health visitor is a nurse with post-registration qualification who provides a continuing service to families and individuals in the community. The work has five main aspects:

1. The prevention of mental, physical and emotional ill health and its consequences.
2. Early detection of ill health and the surveillance of high-risk groups.
3. Recognition and identification of need and mobilization of appropriate resources where necessary.
4. Health teaching.
5. Provision of care; this will include support during periods of stress, and advice and guidance in cases of illness as well as in the care and management of children. The health visitor is not, however, actively engaged in technical nursing procedures.

No other worker at present combines the type of knowledge and skills outlined, and the service the health visitor offers is essential if medicosocial problems are to be contained within manageable proportions in relation to available resources in money and personnel, quite apart from the promotion of the health of the community in its widest sense.

The World Health Organization Technical Report No. 167 states that

public health nursing is a special field of nursing which combines the skills of nursing, public health and some phases of social assistance. It functions as part of the total public health programme for the promotion of health, the improvement of conditions in the social and physical environment, rehabilitation and the prevention of illness and disability.

(Extract from a CETHV leaflet, 1974, revised in 1978)

APPENDIX B
FUNCTIONS OF THE SCHOOL NURSE

A definitive role for the school nurse has yet to be given by the Government Departments, but the following functions were agreed by the Working Group at the time when the syllabus was produced and are based on previous departmental guidelines. They do not preclude the nurse from undertaking such other activities as the employing authority may require.

THE PLACE OF THE SCHOOL NURSE WITHIN THE HEALTH VISITING SERVICE

It is desirable for the school nurse to relate to health visitors at field level, and through them to the Nursing Officer. Wherever possible, health visitors should retain overall responsibility for school health by being allocated a certain number of schools, so that the school nurse can work with these health visitors, and firm links with primary care teams can be established [CNO(77)8]. The expertise of the health visitor will be available in some areas for undertaking certain aspects of school nursing, and in others for advice and support of the school nurse, particularly in advising on health education, and children with social, emotional or physical handicaps. See DHSS Circular HRC/(74)/5.

FUNCTIONS OF THE SCHOOL NURSE (WITHOUT THE HEALTH VISITOR'S CERTIFICATE)

As a member of the school health team, the school nurse should undertake duties in a certain number of schools, and clinic sessions related to school health which may take place outside school premises. The nurse will assume responsibility for delegated work, which may in some areas be undertaken by a health visitor/school nurse, according to the policy of the area concerned and the availability of suitably qualified staff.

Co-operation with the health visitor is necessary to provide links between home, school, and other agencies, in matters relating to the health of the schoolchild. Such co-operation requires the presentation of relevant information on problems to the head-teacher and, in turn, informing the primary care team of any school difficulties.

Co-operation with the clinical medical officer regarding any medical and/or social problems encountered by children is also required.

The school nurse is also expected to be able to:

1. Advise on health matters within the school setting which are within his or her scope and work as a health educator in the widest sense.
2. Participate in health surveys as and when required; these would include the organisation of routine hygiene inspections.
3. Make preparations for medical inspections including the necessary screening procedures, apart from those, such as audiometry, which may be undertaken by technicians.
4. Attend medical inspections in order to facilitate the co-operation of services, and take part in discussion with parents and school doctor as necessary.
5. Arrange and organise immunisation programmes within the school.
6. Attend clinic sessions, related to school health, which may not take place at the school, e.g. at eye clinics and enuretic clinics.
7. In conjunction with the clinical medical officer, follow-up and give health teaching regarding any outbreak of infection.
8. Make arrangements for follow-up home visits, wherever possible in co-operation with the appropriate health visitor, bearing in mind in so doing the functions of the primary care team and other workers involved with the family,

(Quote from CETHV (1977) *Guidelines to a Syllabus for a Course in School Nursing*, November).

APPENDIX C
RECENT JOURNAL ARTICLES

In past years there were few articles referring directly to school nurses or school nursing practice. This appears to have changed dramatically in recent years, demonstrating the increasing value placed on school nurses. The selection given below, although limited and selective, is intended to whet the appetite of the reader. Some articles are of relevance to school nursing practice, others to professional interests mentioned within this text.

Another change is that some of the material is produced by, not only for, school nurses. It seems certain that there are talents still hidden among this professional group, and hopefully more evidence of this will emerge in the foreseeable future.

SCHOOL NURSING

1. Report of the Seminar (unpublished), *Nursing Services to Schools*, held at the NHS Training Centre, Harrogate, in March 1985, by invitation of the DHSS. The report outlines aims for the school nursing service, including flexibility and health advice to education authorities. Conclusions include recommendations about key elements, such as better service planning, concentrating on objectives that are achievable, and the development of reliable measures of effectiveness and performance.
2. School Nurses (1978) *Community Outlook*, October, pp. 289–304. The first magazine supplement to concentrate on articles and reports of interest to this group. Despite the date, few have lost their relevance.

3. School Nurses Supplement (1986) *Health Visitor*, July, pp. 227–233. Some articles by school nurses, and one lengthy study of school meals.
4. An account by K. Fletcher, School Nurse, Hampshire (1985) as yet unpublished, of the *History of the Training of School Nurses*, with particular reference to the currently approved courses.
5. Nash, W. (1985) The day they made contact, *Community Outlook*, May, pp. 14–16. This describes an investigation into how much contact school nurses in Hampshire have with other professionals.
6. Thompson, F. (1986) A health visitor for schools, *Health Visitor*, January, pp. 12–14. A description of the establishment of a schools health visitor post is followed by details of some of the activities and responsibilities entailed.
7. School Nurses Supplement (1986) *Health Visitor*, March. A series of articles and reports of conferences and a useful list of members of the HVA School Nurses Group.
8. The Education Act (1981) *The Role of the Named Person*. Philippa Russell looks at aspects of this role, and suggests a wider definition than is usually found in a school nurse's job specification, including patient/client advocacy and facilitator of parental involvement (Voluntary Council for Handicapped Children – paper circulated 1983).
9. Rustia, J. *et al.* (1984) Redefinition of school nursing practice: Integrating the developmentally disabled, *Journal of School Health*, February, pp. 58–62. This study considers some of the unmet health needs of children and adolescents.
10. Synoground, G. (1984) A programme to prepare prospective school nurses, *Journal of School Health*, September, pp. 295–298.
11. Collis, J. (1985) Why educate school nurses? *Health Visitor*, May, pp. 123–124. This traces the important role school nurses can play in educating parents, teachers and children, and examines the benefits of training courses to achieve this end.
12. Staunton, P. (1985) In a class of their own? *Community Outlook*, September. The author assesses the educational opportunities for school nurses and makes some suggestions for the future.
13. Nash, W. (1986) A position of importance, *Community View*, September. This describes the unique and fundamental role of the school nurse.

PREVENTION IN EDUCATIONAL SETTINGS

1. Report of a seminar held under the auspices of WHO, Regional Office for Europe, received in May 1986. The subject was 'Family Breakdown';

the positive role of nurses and midwives was demonstrated, as well as the effect on children of all ages. Among 25 recommendations the following are most pertinent: much greater emphasis should be placed on primary and secondary prevention (this should include work in schools); nurses and their employers should initiate a campaign to inform the public of their actual and potential role as sources of first-line prevention and support.

2. Measuring is back in fashion (1986) *The British Journal for Nurses in Child Health*, March to July, No. 1–5. A series of valuable articles by different authors, looking at measuring techniques and their value and relevance, as well as some conditions which can be determined by accurate measurements.

3. Catching them early (1985) *Community Outlook*, April. Three articles (one by a school nurse, one by a mother and one by a professor of child health) relating growth disorders and their discovery.

4. Johnson, A. (1986) Screening tests for hearing and visual impairment: how and when are they done? *Health Visitor*, May, pp. 140–144. The importance of variations in techniques is part of this critical appraisal.

5. Shillitoe, R. and Reed, S. (1986) Dry at night, *Community Outlook*, March, pp. 20–23. The authors discuss methods of treatment for enuresis, and the role of health visitors and school nurses.

6. Pratt, L. (1984) Integrating the child with Spina Bifida into school, *Health Visitor*, August, pp. 242. The author, a school nurse, looks at integration and the role of the school nurse.

7. Leenders, F., Orr, J., Peckham, C. and Senturia, Y. (1986) Why we're missing the point, *Nursing Times*, August 20th. Looks at aspects of immunization and the nurse's role within a series of articles.

NURSING ROLES

1. A family snapshot (1986) *Nursing Times*, August. This gives three authors' views of the current situation pertaining in families and society, and suggests nursing roles. Elements of primary, secondary and tertiary prevention in family breakdown situations are indicated, with the need for a multidisciplinary approach.

2. Report of a Working Party of the Society of Nurse Advisers, Child Health (1985) on the implementation of the Education Act, 1981. A survey of intent and achievement to date, containing data provided by health authorities.

3. Probing the practice (1986) *Nursing Times*, April 30th, pp. 47–51. A

series of articles on evaluation, including peer review and quality assurance tools. Although the emphasis is on evaluating nursing care in the ward situation, the principles apply to all branches of nursing, including school nursing.

4. Self-assessment (1986) *Nursing Times,* September 24th (occasional paper). Part of a series on assessing nurses, indicating a range of activities which should be helpful, and providing information on the source of some distance-learning materials.

5. Walton, J. (1986) Lessons from the ombudsman's reports, *Nursing Times,* July 2nd, pp. 54–57. This provides some thought-provoking instances of unsympathetic staff attitudes, failure to keep proper records, increased expectations, clinical judgement and the nurses' position and how the health service commissioner (ombudsman) assesses complaints.

6. Dainow, S. (1986) Believe in yourself, *Nursing Times,* July 2nd, pp. 49–51. This discusses how assertiveness techniques can benefit every nurse (part of a series).

7. Darbyshire, P., Meerabeau, L. and Watson, C. (1986) Is a mother's place in the home? *Nursing Times,* June 4th, pp. 28–35. A series of articles considering some of the myths of motherhood, nurses as parents and employment legislation, motherhood and nursing and single mothers. Relevant for many school nurses who combine professional roles with those of parenthood.

8. Wells, R., Pyne, R. and Melia, K. (1986) Informed consent – the great conspiracy, *Nursing Times,* May 21st, pp. 22–27. A series of articles exploring aspects of the nurse's duty, the implications in terms of professional conduct and some of the moral issues.

9. Watkins, M. (1986) Strength through unity, *Community Outlook,* March, pp. 29–31. The author considers that a unified, political approach from all community nurses is the only way forward.

10. Smith, S. (1985) Political animals, *Community Outlook,* December, pp. 7–10. The author explains why she believes primary health care nurses must become political, and suggests some ideas on how to go about it.

11. Hyland, M. and Frapwell, C. (1986) Afraid to tell, *Nursing Times,* October 1st, pp. 50–51. The authors examine the psychological implications of professional misconduct. They consider the anxiety over standards among those responsible for commenting on other's malpractice.

HEALTH PROMOTION AND HEALTH EDUCATION

1. Greene, A. and MacFarlane, A. (1985) Parent-held child record cards – a

comparison of types; and Pearson, P. (1985) Parent-held records – what parents think, *Health Visitor, 58*, January. The research was based on a doctor/health visitor caseload, and includes school health elements. Though inconclusive, these articles could point the way towards future practice.

2. Huxley-Robinson, M. (1985) Counselling the bereaved child – the role of the school nurse, *Health Visitor, 58*, pp. 253–255. The author, a school nursing sister, considers the profound and longstanding effects of bereavement on young children, and discusses the role of the school nurse in aiding children to overcome these effects.

3. Cliff, K.S. (1985) Health promotion: can the nursing profession influence policies? *Midwife, Health Visitor and Community Nurse, 21*, September, pp. 302–309. This article is written from a limited, medical viewpoint relating to specific incidents and incidence, but it challenges the assumption that nurses are better informed than the general public. The latter point deserves closer consideration.

4. Reports of the HVA Conference (1985) *Health Visitor*, January. 'Professional challenges in health visiting and school nursing', including 'The re-emergence of nutrition and its role in health'.

5. Gay, M. (1986) Drug and solvent abuse in adolescents, *Nursing Times*, January 29th, pp. 34–35. The author discusses the importance of co-operation among community agencies in managing the problem.

6. Walker, C. (1986) The fats of life, *Nursing Times*, May 7th, pp. 20–21. This article looks at the implications of a hitherto suppressed government report on the nutritional content of schoolchildren's diet.

7. Hunt, S. (1985) Below the breadline, *Community Outlook*, October. This explains why the NACNE diet is not feasible for those on the breadline, and explodes a few myths in the process.

8. Richardson, J. (1985) Eat yourself healthier, *Nursing Mirror*, May 22nd, pp. 16–18. The author reports on a campaign to create greater awareness of a healthy diet, including the reaction of school 'tuck' shops and some teaching materials.

9. Catrone, C. and Siebert Sadler, L. (1984) A developmental model for teenage parent education. *Journal of School Health, 54* (No. 2), February, pp. 63–67. The authors look at providing education for teenage parents.

10. Strehlow, M.S. (1986) Iatrogenesis in Health Education, *Health Visitor, 59*, May, pp. 148–149. A brief outline is given of the possible dangers and pitfalls of health education.

CHILD ABUSE

1. Holmes, P. (1986) It's OK to say no, *Nursing Times,* January 15th, pp. 17–18. The author reviews a new book that puts the message about resisting child abuse across in a lively way.
2. Evans, R. (1985) The silent victims, *Nursing Times,* November 27th, pp. 59–60. This article considers a range of typical signs which should set alarm bells ringing about child abuse.
3. Trowell, J. (1985) Working with families where incest is actual or feared, *Health Visitor, 58,* July, pp. 189–193. This article describes the main forms of incest and sexual abuse within families, using examples from the author's experience to illustrate the kind of problems that can be encountered and the ways of dealing with them.
4. Frude, N. (1986) Sexual abuse of children, *Midwife, Health Visitor and Community Nurse,* pp. 302–304. The author looks at the evidence which appears to show that serious psychological damage of victims can be avoided.

RELEVANT MISCELLANY

1. Vousden, M. (1986) Mind your language, *Nursing Times,* August 20th, pp. 35. The author emphasizes the importance of choosing words carefully (a series of three articles).
2. White, J. (1986) School non-attenders and long-term problems, *Midwife, Health Visitor and Community Nurse, 22,* June, pp. 190–191. This looks at truancy, school refusal and phobia among 1 per cent of primary and 10 per cent of secondary schoolchildren.
3. Darbyshire, P. (1986) Can Tiger come too? *Nursing Times,* April 2nd, pp. 40–42. The author discusses why so may children feel a need to develop their own fantasy world.
4. Williams, B. (1986) Attacking fleas, *British Journal for Nurses in Child Health,* August, *1* (No. 6), pp. 184–186. The author looks at the habitat of vermin, and their happiness at finding themselves in luxurious, carpeted and centrally heated homes.
5. Clemenson, C. (1986) Boys and girls come out to play? *Nursing Times,* February. This highlights the lessons for school nurses within the government guidelines on AIDS.
6. Foster, J. *et al.* (1986) A child's view, *Nursing Times,* September. A survey of young people's attitudes to mental illness revealed surprisingly compassionate feelings.

7. Holden, H. and Fogelman, K. (1978) *Health and Illness in the National Child Development Study*; some findings from the 11-year and 16-year sweeps (1969–1974), National Children's Bureau.

8. National Children's Bureau (1984) Teenage parents – a review of research, Highlight No. 59, February.

9. *Education – New Deal for Children with Special Needs*. Factsheets. Centre for Studies on Integration in Education, The Spastics Society, 12 Park Crescent, London W1N 4EQ.

10. *The Danger Overhead. Childright No. 31*, October 1986. 'Fluorescent lighting is cheap, efficient and lasts longer than ordinary lighting. The problem is it might also be dangerous to children because of the materials used in its manufacture, the radiation it emits and the glare it creates.' This article examines the growing body of evidence, including warning leaflets published by the Health and Safety Executive during 1986, and the guidelines contained in Education (School Premises) Regulations and Education (Schools and Further Education) Regulations issued by the DES in 1981.

11. Sutherland, M. and Fasko, D. (1984) Compentencies of Florida school health educators, *Journal of School Health, 54* (No. 9), September, pp. 358–359.

12. Frick, S. (1985) School Nursing in Great Britain, *Journal of School Health*, 55 (No. 3), March, pp. 120–122. The author is from the university of South Carolina, and gives her impression of the British scene.

13. Shapiro, R. (1985) Taking precautions, *Nursing Times*, February 27th, pp. 20–21. The author examines the measures nurses are now taking to stay within the law.

14. Hadley, A. (1985) Lessons of a tragedy, *Nursing Times*, July 17th, pp. 17–18. The author talks to a school nurse who was caught up in the aftermath of the St Albans coach crash which killed five children.

APPENDIX D
DEFINITION OF CASE AND WORKLOAD

CASELOAD

A school nursing caseload is the population for which the nurse has a designated responsibility. It could be based on a geographically defined catchment area and/or specific school or other institution populations.

Although not necessarily involved with all of the population on a frequent contact basis, the responsibility for the whole population as defined by the employing authority is ongoing. This approach is comparable with general medical practitioner and health visitor caseloads for which there is a continual responsibility, but not all clients are seen on a regular basis. This concept of caseload differs from that of district nurses and social workers where the caseload is usually reckoned to be the number of cases for whom they have a specific responsibility at a particular point in time.

WORKLOAD

The workload encompasses the whole range of activities for which the nurse has professional responsibility. This includes work with all those individuals and groups with whom the nurse is in professional contact, the identification of health needs within the caseload, and planning and implementing appropriate responses. It also includes participating in activities related to developments within health and associated services.

INDEX